Ethics and Midwifery

Issues in Contemporary Practice

Edited by

Lucy Frith BA MPhil

Lecturer in Health Care Ethics,
Department of Primary Care,
The University of Liverpool, UK

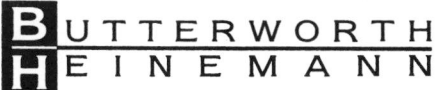

Butterworth-Heinemann
Linacre House, Jordan Hill, Oxford OX2 8DP
A division of Reed Educational and Professional Publishing Ltd

Ɽ A member of the Reed Elsevier plc group

OXFORD   BOSTON   JOHANNESBURG
MELBOURNE   NEW DELHI   SINGAPORE

First published 1996

British Library Cataloguing in Publication Data
'Ethics and midwifery: issues in contemporary practice'
   1 Obstetrics – Moral and ethical aspects
   I Frith, Lucy
   174.2

ISBN 0 7506 3056 6

Library of Congress Cataloguing in Publication Data
Ethics and midwifery: issues in contemporary practice/edited by Lucy Frith.
   p. cm.
   Includes bibliographical references and index.
   ISBN 0 7506 3056 6
   1 Obstetrics – Moral and ethical aspects. 2 Midwifery – Moral and ethical
   aspects. I Frith, Lucy.
   RG526.E84   96–25888
   174'.2 – dc20   CIP

Typeset by Latimer Trend & Company Ltd, Plymouth
Printed and bound in Great Britain by Biddles Ltd,
Guildford and King's Lynn

Contents

List of Contributors

Karen Bartter, MA, RGN, RM, ADM, Cert. Ed
Senior Lecturer in Midwifery, University of Wolverhampton

Rachel Clarke, MA, (Medical Ethics), RM, ADM, MTD/Cert.Ed
Lecturer in Midwifery Studies, School of Nursing and Midwifery,
University of East Anglia

Soo Downe, BA, RM, MSc
Research Midwife, Derby City General Hospital NHS Trust

Heather Draper, BA, MA, PhD
Lecturer in Biomedical Ethics, University of Birmingham

Lucy Frith, BA, MPhil
Lecturer in Health Care Ethics, Department of Primary Care, The
University of Liverpool

Carolyn Hicks, BA, MA, PhD, PGCE, CPsychol
Senior Lecturer in Psychology, University of Birmingham

Janet Holt, MPhil, BA, PGDipE, RGN, RM, ADM, RNT
Lecturer in Nursing, School of Health Care Studies, University of Leeds

David Lamb, BA, PhD
Honorary Reader in Bioethics, Department of Biomedical Science and
Bioethics, University of Birmingham

Helen Lewison, MA(Oxon)
National Childbirth Trust Antenatal Teacher and Adviser on National
Childbirth Trust Maternity Services Committee

Rosemary Mander, MSc, PhD, RGN, SCM, MTD
Senior Lecturer, Department of Nursing Studies, University of Edinburgh

v

Hazel McHaffie, PhD, SRN, SCM
Research Fellow, Institute of Medical Ethics, Department of Medicine,
University of Edinburgh

Pam Miller, BA, SRN, SCM, Dip.N, Cert.Ed
Senior Midwife, Neonatal Unit, Birmingham Women's Hospital

Jane Pritchard, BA(Hons)
Solicitor. Currently Research Assistant in Professional Ethics. Registered
for MPhil/PhD

Jean Proud, BA, MSc, SRN, SCM, MTD
Midwife Teacher, St Martins College, Lancaster

Catherine Williams, SRN, HVCert, SCM, BA(Hons)
Lecturer in Women's Health, Department of Primary Health Care,
University College of St Martin, Lancaster

Introduction

The aim of this book is to consider some of the main ethical issues and dilemmas that midwives face in practice that have received relatively little coverage in mainstream ethical literature. Midwives have had to use textbooks written for other health care professionals (HCP), and have had to find a wide range of books and articles to obtain material on all areas of their practice. This book brings together some of the many topics that are of relevance to the midwife and provides a starting point for midwives who are considering the ethical aspects of their practice. Throughout the book midwives will be referred to as 'she' and this is used to encompass all midwives.

In this introduction I want to consider some general issues relating to the relationship between midwifery and ethics, to look at why a separate collection on midwifery ethics is needed and why ethics is invaluable to HCP in their everyday roles.

There have been many books written about both medical and nursing ethics and it might be asked, 'Why is a specific collection on midwifery ethics needed?' The answer to this is two fold. First, the structure of midwifery as a profession is changing, as proposed by *Changing Childbirth* (Department of Health, 1993) and second, because of the distinctive type of client that midwives work with. These issues will be considered in this introduction, concluding with an outline of the contents of this collection.

The relevance of ethics to midwifery and health care practice

The claim that ethics is important not only to midwives but all HCP has often been disputed and I want to consider this initially before moving on to demonstrate why midwifery ethics merits separate consideration. There are those who would argue that ethics serves little purpose to any HCP in any form. There is not space in this introduction to examine all aspects of this claim (for a discussion of this see Lamb, 1995) and I will concentrate on advancing the position that ethics is essential to good clinical practice and, therefore, is relevant to all health care practice.

If the midwife is the lead professional in the majority of 'low-risk' births then she is responsible for all decisions made in relation to her client and this incorporates a degree of moral responsibility for these decisions. To be an able practitioner means that not only must she be clinically knowledgeable and keep this knowledge updated but also that she has an understanding of the ethical issues that surround maternity care. She must function as a clinically sound and ethical practitioner, for the two go hand-in-hand. This book gives a broad overview of some of the kinds of ethical problems that midwives may face in their practice. It demonstrates that there is an ethical dimension in all clinical decisions (however large or small) and that the midwife needs to be acquainted with these dimensions so that she can provide the highest standard of care and give an adequate justification for any action she undertakes.

It is necessary to substantiate the claim that there is an ethical dimension to all clinical decisions, and that further, a good clinician is an ethical one. I will consider two points to support this. First, by the nature of medicine and midwifery it can be argued that these are professions that have certain ethical goals as their fundamental aim. The fundamental aim of medicine is to promote health in order to enable people to live fulfilled lives; the choice of this aim is an ethical decision based on notions of helping and caring for others in times of physical and mental distress. Daryl Koehn in *The Ground of Professional Ethics* (1994) states, 'professions are . . . inherently ethical practices'. The point here is not to go into an extended discussion of what constitutes a profession but simply to claim that HCP seek to provide a genuine good to their clientele and what constitutes this good is an ethical decision. A genuine good in this context is something we want for its own sake, i.e. health, justice, as opposed to wealth that we want as a way of getting other things. Hence, by fulfilling one's professional obligations as a health carer one is already engaged in the pursuit of an ethical goal. Clinical procedures are the means by which we fulfil certain goals, not the goals themselves (which might be a return to health, increased autonomy, etc.), and these goals are determined by ethical criteria.

The second point to justify my claim is that often the appropriate course of action is conceived in terms of what is the clinically acceptable thing to do and what are the clinical demands of the situation. However, it is only in very rare cases that there is no debate over the clinically correct course of action and further, since the decision concerns another human being, what is appropriate for that individual is almost always a value judgement. This is particularly prevalent in the area of childbirth where the woman (in uncomplicated births) has many realistic clinical options available to her.

To illustrate this consider the following case study. A woman decides that she wishes to have a home birth and the community midwife readily agrees. However, after a routine antenatal visit at 35 weeks it becomes apparent that the baby is in the breech position. After the ultrasound it is determined that the baby is a good size for the number of weeks and is unlikely to move. The midwife now advises the woman that the home birth might not be such a good idea. However, the woman is reluctant to accept the midwife's advice, stating that breech births used to be routinely delivered at home and insists on a home birth. What should the midwife do? There are two elements to the midwife's assessment of the situation, the clinical and the ethical. The breech presentation indicates risk factors that might be better managed in a hospital. These are clinical reasons. However, these have to be weighed up against the woman's autonomous decision to direct her care. This is an ethical consideration. Here the conflict is between respecting the woman's autonomy and trying to promote what is beneficial for her and the baby. When coming to a decision as to whether the midwife should push her earlier recommendation, both clinical and ethical factors will come into play. Hence, it is important to see ethics as essential to good clinical practice. This is reflected in the General Medical Council's *Duties of a Doctor* (1995), which replaces the 'Blue Book' as a guide for doctors on their professional duties. *Duties of a Doctor* views observance of ethical obligations as a crucial aspect of good medical practice and not something subsidiary to clinical factors.

Why midwifery ethics needs separate consideration

I shall now outline why, in my view, midwifery ethics merits separate consideration, by looking at the changing structure of the midwifery profession and the distinctive concerns that motivate practice and delineate what midwifery is. These distinctive elements need to be reflected in the ethical consideration. Further, as midwifery is an independent profession it is imperative that the ethical literature reflects the dynamics of actual midwifery practice. It is important not to separate such ethical consideration from the practical context, as this could make it less immediately relevant for practitioners.

The midwifery profession

The professional status of midwifery is rapidly changing (Department of Health, 1993) and the structure of child-bearing in Britain could be radically different in the next century. It will be based on new principles of care which stress respect for individual autonomy. Care must now be 'women-centred' in that, 'The woman should be able to make her decision about the plan for birth ... [and] feel confident that these professionals will respect her right to choose her care' (Department of Health, 1993). The midwife in many instances will be, 'the lead professional—undertaking the key role in the planning and provision of care' (1993). By taking on this role midwives will have increased professional responsibility for their clients. Moreover, 'Maternity service should be readily and easily accessible to all. They should be sensitive to the needs of the local population and based primarily in the community' (Department of Health, 1993). Women-centred community care, with a midwife as lead professional will mean that midwives, more than ever, will be responsible for not only making decisions about the management of pregnancies, but also for ensuring that the woman's wishes and choices are respected. To aim to encourage patient choice is clearly an ethical imperative that is justified by appealing to theories of personal autonomy (autonomy literally means self-governance). In implementing the recommendations of *Changing Childbirth* (Department of Health, 1993), a degree of ethical sophistication is required from practitioners. The changing role of the midwife, the increased decision-making capacity (giving the midwife more professional and ethical responsibility for the patient) and the imperative to increase patient choice mean that midwives will, increasingly, need a grounding in ethics to enable them adequately to provide this new form of maternity care.

The distinctive concerns of midwifery

Although it would be almost impossible to divide the HCP into watertight compartments with no overlap whatsoever, there are different *overriding* concerns that inform and motivate each professional group. Daryl Koehn makes this point (1994) when she addresses the concept of what it is to be a professional, 'each of these practices has its own special ethic, one deriving its peculiar and distinctive character'. HCP all have certain fundamental elements of their practice in common, such as caring, diagnosing and treating, but doctors, nurses and midwives place different emphasis and importance on each element. For instance, for the medical profession the emphasis is placed on diagnostic skills and treatment regimens, while for the nursing profession the emphasis is on caring, support and the ability to interpret the doctors' treatment plans. Midwives, however, have slightly different concerns, although they incorporate all of the aforementioned elements into their practice. Midwives' clients are usually healthy and experiencing a life-changing event of huge magnitude. For this reason the midwives' client group can often be radically different from those with which most HCP come into contact. This client group needs a very different kind of service from those patients who are in some way 'ill', although with the increasing emphasis on health promotion this reduces the close link between doctors and disease/illness management.

It can be said that midwives are required to be more than good clinicians and carers (in the usual health care sense), as Lesley Page (1995) puts it, 'The midwife must be more than a clinician, she must also be a companion, a skilled companion. . . . Our work is concerned with supporting parents in their adaptation to parenthood, as much as with providing physical care'. In this way, midwives have both different care strategies and different ends to other HCP. The midwives' care strategy can be one of facilitating genuine choice (as the woman is not sick and in this respect her autonomy is not compromised by ill health) and making the experience as pleasant as possible. A woman's experience of birth can affect the way she feels and adapts to motherhood, so it is important that this is as rewarding an experience as possible. Birth is not an unpleasant means to an end in the same way an operation is, which is performed as a necessary evil and something one expects to cause discomfort. Midwives also have different ends for their practice; their goal is not to cure but to help facilitate a natural event and to prepare their client for parenthood and a future change in lifestyle.

Midwives are in a good position to facilitate client choice, as proposed by *Changing Childbirth* (Department of Health, 1993), and this requirement demands a degree of ethical knowledge in order to transfer this blanket assertion into a practical strategy. One of the main problems with facilitating choice comes when choices conflict or the midwife feels the client is choosing an option that is detrimental to her welfare. Here the clash is between the client's wish for self-determination and the midwife's perception of the client's best interests. A client's choices can also be restricted by limited care options being available (i.e. due to scarce resources) or by the client's lack of understanding of what could be offered. In weighing up all these competing elements the midwife has to employ a sophisticated understanding of the ethical issues. This volume examines the issue of choice in detail and addresses the difficult ethical dilemmas that arise when the choices of different individuals conflict.

Due to the distinctive concerns of midwifery practice, midwives need to focus on those aspects of ethics that relate closely to their practice, i.e. the promotion of autonomy and facilitating choice. This is not to say that these elements are not present in other HCP practice, rather it is a matter of degree and what each profession takes as its main focus.

It is also useful for midwives to be presented with case studies and issues that they face directly in their own practice. Many cases that are used in nursing ethics texts are simply not relevant to midwives. There are some general themes in all health care ethics, such as autonomy, beneficence, etc., and these could be discussed in relation to general case studies. However, there are very different manifestations of the problems of patient autonomy created by caring, for example, for an incompetent elderly man, than those midwives face in their practice and these subtle differences can be immeasurably important in actual practice. Case studies need to be situation-based so that they can be of maximum use to midwives. Further, some of the most difficult ethical dilemmas midwives face are unique to their sphere of practice. A prime example is the potential conflict between a woman and the fetus. The issues raised by these circumstances cannot be replicated by other situations. Thus, specific case presentations enable midwives to see the relevance of ethics more clearly and apply it to their own experiences.

To turn now to the role of ethics in midwifery education. Ethics is now part of the professional training of many health carers. With the increase in ethics courses in HCP training, the question has been asked, 'What is being achieved by such an inclusion?' Are we implying that student midwives are not moral beings and need to be coached into behaving morally? (For a discussion of this issue see Hunt, 1994.) I do not think this is the implication, rather the inclusion of ethics is an attempt to give students the forum to consider difficult cases in the safe environment of the classroom with ample time before they encounter them in practice. Just as we give student midwives the opportunity to consider theory and to practise clinical skills before performing them on an actual client, the same opportunity should be afforded to the practice of ethical skills so that costly mistakes can be avoided.

Further, the disciplines of ethics and philosophy are, what is frequently called in education, transferable skills. The process of setting out the problem, distinguishing its component parts, providing careful and adequate definitions and formulating a logical argument, are the main jobs of the philosopher. These skills can be applied to other areas to enable the HCP better to perform her duties; for instance, such skills are invaluable in writing essays or reports, they aid the ability to put forward a reasoned argument, help clarify the salient issues and uncover sources of disagreement. In this way the ethical process can be a useful resource in education programmes.

This introduction has attempted to indicate why there is a need for a separate consideration of midwifery ethics and the practical relevance of ethics in general. I shall now give an outline and rationale of the contents of this book.

Outline of the contents

The central themes of this collection are autonomy and choice. *Changing Childbirth* (Department of Health, 1993) has stipulated that maternity care should be women-centred and so the promoting of client choice and autonomy is rapidly becoming a central concern of providers of maternity care. Not only this, with midwives often as the lead professionals, the professional status and autonomy of midwives are also coming under increasing scrutiny. This book considers the issues of choice and autonomy from both the clients' and the midwives' perspectives. Clearly, in an ideal world individuals' choices would not conflict and the freedom to choose would be straightforward. However, in practice one of the most common ways in which choices are restricted is when they clash with another's choice to do differently (i.e. the midwife and the woman in the case study are involved in such a conflict).

The chapters give a broad overview of the many ethical problems that midwives could face in practice. It is not intended to be an introduction to moral theory, rather it raises issues in their practical context to demonstrate the tensions and conflicts that exist, enabling realistic solutions and approaches to be formulated.

The volume is divided into three sections, Everyday Issues, Technological Issues and Professional Issues, and points are cross-referenced throughout the chapters so that links can be made. Inevitably some subjects will not be covered and some views not expressed. One volume cannot possibly cover all the problematic situations midwives might face, but ways of approaching problems are indicated and can be applied to those issues not raised.

The first section, Everyday Issues, examines in detail some of the ethical problems that arise in everyday midwifery practice, focusing particularly on the difficulties that are created by conflicting choices. Heather Draper considers the general issue of consent in childbirth in Chapter 1. This chapter gives a broad introduction to the issue of consent, discussing the theoretical basis of the doctrine. She then goes on to consider the practical importance of consent and examines the possible conflicts that could arise if the mother refuses consent for treatment that might be in the best interests of the fetus. This chapter introduces the subsequent discussions on consent.

In Chapter 2 Helen Lewison examines choices in childbirth and highlights areas of conflict. The issues are considered from the perspective of the women using the maternity services, one that the author points out is often under-represented. As a user representative for the maternity services (NCT) Helen Lewison is particularly able to voice these concerns. The chapter uses the East Herts Trust dispute (1993) over water births as a case study and explores the fundamental importance for maternity services of informed choice and demonstrates the ethical importance of each individual exercising autonomy. The chapter concludes with recommendations for the extension of choice in maternity services, at both national and local level, by extensive consultation with users and all other interested groups.

Chapter 3 extends the discussion about consent to specific clinical interventions in labour, focusing primarily on epidural analgesia in uncomplicated labour. Rosemary Mander considers the likelihood of two salient features of consent (information and voluntariness) being feasible in the context of epidural analgesia and other interventions in labour such as Caesarean section and episiotomy. She concludes that the acceptance of epidural services has been fostered by the expectation that mothers will fail to cope with the pain of uncomplicated labour and that further research is needed into pain control, so that such a service can be provided on an ethical basis.

Chapter 4 considers another intervention in pregnancy, that of ultrasound. Jean Proud looks at the ethical dilemmas that are raised by routine screening by ultrasound, considering the problem of obtaining informed consent for the procedure, the often paternalistic attitudes of health carers, the importance of truth telling and the right of women to direct their own treatment. The chapter argues that women must be kept informed at all stages of the screening process and screening should only be carried out by proficient and up-to-date practitioners.

Chapters 5 and 6 broaden the discussion to cover general underlying themes of relevance to all pregnancy and childbirth. These chapters address philosophical aspects of the childbirth, i.e. the underlying theories of how it is conceptualized and they elaborate on the ethical and practical dimensions of adopting these theoretical positions. In Chapter 5 Soo Downe examines the concept of normality. Midwives are trained to be experts in normal childbirth and any deviation from the norm must be referred to a medical practitioner. With the advent of new ways of working, such as the lead professional role, it becomes important to have a clear idea about what is meant by normality. This is a debate in which midwives should take the lead and formulate a definition of normality based on good research and practical evidence. Soo Downe considers definitions of abnormality and risk, the effects such definitions have on pregnant women and the professional implications for midwives.

This section concludes with Catherine Williams' consideration of the relationship between sexuality, the reproductive continuum and the midwife. The increasing medicalization of childbirth has separated sexuality from the birth process and reduced midwives to coy maiden birth attendants. Catherine Williams argues that if sexuality is excluded from the birth process, rather than making it safer, it actually complicates and confuses the relationship between the midwife and mother. By conceptualizing birth as a medical event the diversity of women's needs are not recognized, forcing women into experiencing birth in a predetermined way. She claims that midwives need to recognize and acknowledge the sexual nature of childbirth in order to be able to relate honestly to, and support, the person seeking professional assistance.

The second section, Technological Issues, examines some of the ethical dilemmas created by technological interventions in pregnancy. Some of the issues raised in this section will have a direct bearing on midwifery practice, others will be of more general interest so that midwives can be kept informed of the wider ethical issues raised by reproduction.

Chapter 7 considers the ethical issues raised in neonatal intensive care. Pam Miller considers questions such as, should every live-born baby be offered full intensive care and how should this decision be reached, what should be the criteria for withdrawing care and how should babies with congenital abnormalities be managed. Finally, the problem of resources and staffing is addressed and Miller concludes that each practitioner must develop their own ethical stance on the issues raised so that they can provide the best possible care for their patients.

Chapter 8 takes up points briefly considered in Proud's, Miller's and Downes' chapters and focuses on the problem of what should happen if an abnormality is detected by a scan. Janet Holt considers the wider issues raised by screening, looking at questions such as, should people have the choice over what kind of baby they have and the implications of genetic screening for the individual and society. Finally, she considers if such screening has eugenic implications and whether this is immoral and therefore to be avoided.

In Chapter 9 David Lamb considers the leading arguments for and against the use of fetal tissue transplantation, building on the discussion of abortion developed in Holt's chapter. The separation principle is exemplified, according to which the alleged benefits of fetal transplantation can be separated from what some people see as the stigma of voluntary abortion. The chapter looks at the issue of who should consent for the transplants and examines how the fetus is conceptualized. The chapter concludes with recommendations for safeguards under which fetal tissue transplants could be performed ethically.

In Chapter 10 I examine reproductive technologies and aim to give the reader a broad introduction to the ethical problems raised by assisted conception techniques. I consider the legislative provisions and outline the main ethical problems that these techniques have raised. The chapter concludes with an indication of practical ethical difficulties that pregnancies conceived in this way can create for the midwife involved in their management.

The final section, Professional Issues, concentrates on the possible constraints on midwives' professional autonomy and considers the codes of practice and the professional obligations that delineate midwifery practice. Part 3 also examines the ethics of research as this is increasingly becoming part of midwives' professional obligations to ensure that practice is research-based. Chapter 11 looks at codes of practice and how these can be used to inform ethical judgements about practical situations. The role of codes in delineating professions and the issue of midwifery as a profession are considered. Jane Pritchard argues that to make the code more effective education is needed to enable practitioners to have the relevant abilities to make decisions about what course of action is ethically correct. Only with this accompanying education can midwives be expected to make ethically competent and justifiable decisions in a clinical context.

Chapter 12 provides a more critical view of the codes of practice and Rachel Clarke argues that the code of professional conduct is unjust in its expectations, as it assumes that midwives are autonomous practitioners when in practice they are unable to exercise such autonomy. Rachel Clarke contends that the contrast between the myth of professional freedom and the observed control of midwives by employers, medicine and the State exposes the fallibility of the midwife's belief about her status in twentieth century child-bearing. Rachel Clarke claims that the code, in assuming such professional autonomy, encourages midwives to make autonomous judgements but punishes them if they do in fact act autonomously.

Chapter 13 considers another aspect of midwifery autonomy and asks if it is possible for the midwife to act as the patient's advocate.

Karen Bartter considers whether it is possible for midwives to carry out this function and outlines the constraints that may reduce her ability to act as advocate. The chapter presents the findings of a research project, undertaken by the author, testing the contention that midwives felt unprepared for their role as advocate and were unable to defend the rights of women to other NHS professionals and those outside the NHS. Karen Bartter concludes that midwives do not have a full understanding of their role as advocate.

The final two chapters focus on the issue of research. Chapter 14 gives a broad introduction to the ethical problems raised by conducting a research project and offers practical advice on elements that should be considered when formulating an ethical research proposal. Carolyn Hicks considers the ethical aspects of issues such as: What is the research topic? Who is to conduct the research? Who will benefit from the research? Where will the research be conducted? How will the participants be treated? How will the research be carried out? How will the findings be disseminated? Chapter 15 develops in more detail some of the issues addressed in the previous chapter and considers the possible ethical problems raised by the researcher holding sensitive information. Hazel McHaffie introduces the problems, such as maintaining confidentiality and handling distressing information, by citing examples taken from her own research experience. The chapter gives clinicians an idea of the constraints upon researchers as well as alerting would-be researchers to some of the possible pitfalls.

Although this book cannot give definitive answers to the ethical dilemmas and tensions encountered in practice, by raising such issues and engaging in discussion, progress towards consensus and resolution can be hastened. An open discussion of these issues can alleviate the isolation many practitioners feel when confronted with ethical problems. By such a discussion the thought processes and reasons for acting can be revealed and opened up to scrutiny so that bad practice can be eliminated and good practice applauded.

Lucy Frith

References

Department of Health (1993). *Changing Childbirth*. HMSO.
General Medical Council (1995). *Duties of a Doctor*. GMC.

Hunt, G. (ed.) (1994). Introduction. In *Ethical Issues in Nursing*. Routledge.

Koehn, D. (1994). *The Ground of Professional Ethics*. Routledge.

Lamb, D. (1995). Introduction. *Treatment Abatement and Withdrawing Therapy*. Avebury.

Page, L. (ed.) (1995). Putting principles in practice. In *Effective Group Practice in Midwifery*, pp. 12–31. Blackwell Science Ltd.

Part One

Everyday Issues

Chapter 1

Consent in childbirth

Heather Draper

Introduction

This chapter looks first at consent from an ethical rather than a legal point of view. It then examines some of the circumstances under which gaining or respecting consent can cause ethical problems for midwives.

Consent as an expression of autonomy

Giving consent prior to any health care procedure is a vital expression of the patient's autonomy. The principle of autonomy is underpinned by two contrasting ideas from moral theory. The first is that autonomy is inextricably linked to responsibility. If I *choose* to do this thing rather than that, then I can, and should, be held responsible for my decision. Likewise, if I am *forced* to do this rather than that, then it would be unfair to hold me responsible for an action over which I had no control: I did not make the decision, it was made for me. Where autonomous choice is exercised, responsibility follows. The same is true of consent. When I consent to some medical or surgical procedure, this is both an expression of my responsibility for myself and also means that I have to take responsibility for the course of action chosen: I cannot blame others for the consequences. The freedom and ability to exercise my autonomy is a necessary condition for me to be considered a moral agent. The second reason to respect autonomy is based on the contention that without individual autonomy there can be no individual innovation, and without individual innovation society would stagnate. Just as the first justification rests upon the assumption that personal responsibility is possible and the exercising of autonomy a good thing, so this justification rests on the assumption that living in society is a good thing and that to remain good, societies must adapt and change. It might seem strange to question what seem to be two fundamentally important things. However, philosophers have indeed questioned whether in reality we have such a thing as free will, whilst politicians have, not infrequently, suggested that benevolent dictatorship might produce the most stable society.

Consent is also a safeguard for the patient's best interests. It is not unreasonable to assume that, given the choice, individuals will only choose to do that which is best for them and, moreover, that they are in the best position to define precisely what that is. However, as Gillon (1986) points out, resting the justification for respecting consent on best interests can create problems. It suggests that the primary concern is not that the patient is granted autonomy but rather that her best interests are served: this is the end for which consent is the means. So, if I insist on a course of action which apparently works against my best interests, then the reason for respecting my wishes has been undermined. If my best interests are those that my carers are seeking to promote, then this end may actually be more effectively achieved by taking a decision on my behalf, by taking the decision out of my hands. One standard response to this conclusion is to argue that best interests can only be determined by the individual concerned, that she alone is the judge of what is best for her.

Ultimately, then, to determine one's position on the value of consent, one has to determine the extent to which one values autonomy. Does one hold it to be absolutely valuable (i.e. nothing can override it) or just relatively valuable (i.e. that there are other more important considerations that can arise)? The former view commits one to allowing the patient always to have the final say (whatever the consequences for her might be). The latter leaves one with the problem of determining which things one values over autonomy and doing so consistently.

Consent and pregnant patients

For pregnant women, midwives and obstetricians there is, however, a further dimension to the giving and receiving of consent. The discussion up to this point assumes that there is one patient making a decision for herself. In the case of pregnant women, this is not so obviously the case as one (or more) fetuses is also involved. For the woman concerned, this issue might be resolved with reference to some view about the status of the fetus. She might feel that until the fetus is born it has no independent moral status and therefore no interests. Alternatively she might believe that the fetus has interests in the future but that these can be outweighed by her own immediate interests (including, perhaps, her interest in her existing family and commitments). Perhaps she may feel that as the mother of this dependant child she must act always in the best interests of that child. However, the position for midwives and obstetricians is even less clear. Not only might the individual practitioner have a view about the status of the fetus which is different from that of her pregnant patient, but she has the additional problem of determining who her patient is, the pregnant woman or the unborn fetus.

Health care workers are charged only and always to act in the best interests of their patients, but if the fetus is also considered to be a patient, then in midwifery (as indeed in other areas of practice) it is possible for there to be a direct conflict of interests between patients and therefore between the duties to those patients. Traditionally, those specializing in midwifery and obstetrics have considered that both the woman and the fetus are patients. However, this dual-patient view is not as obvious in the new speciality of fetal medicine, where the direct object of attention is the fetus rather than the woman. While all practitioners have to respect the autonomy of their pregnant patients, concerns have been raised about how this autonomy can and should be affected by the existence of the unborn fetus. The fetus is clearly not autonomous and is unable to express a point of view. Some carers nevertheless believe that whilst they have a duty to respect the autonomy of the pregnant patient, they must also safeguard the interests of the vulnerable fetus. This conflict will be explored in greater detail later in this chapter in the section: Limits to autonomy.

What constitutes consent?

With the emergence of defensive practice, a greater concern for ethical practice and a change in the dynamics between principal carers have influenced our understanding of what it means both to gain and give consent to therapy. In the past, the doctor was considered to know best and consent was less than a mere formality. Then emerged the idea of informed consent where it was held that the patient should be aware of the risks of and alternatives to any intervention. This was refined to the description of informed and voluntary consent in which information and lack of coercion played a part. More recently, Culver and Gert (1982) introduced the notion of valid consent which highlighted the problems of ensuring that the patient is competent. The trend now is to refer simply to 'consent', which is understood to contain all these elements. Consent must, therefore, be understood with reference to the following four components:

(1) voluntariness;
(2) information;
(3) competence;
(4) decision.

This forms a useful checklist for the practitioner.

Voluntariness

If an act is voluntary it is one that one has chosen for oneself without coercion. Clearly, though, the extent to which an action is voluntary also depends upon how much information was received, whether or not one was deceived and also upon one's ability to decide for oneself. However, it is fruitful for an understanding of consent, that 'voluntariness' in the sense of 'free from coercion' is examined in isolation from information and competence.

Coercion tends to be associated with threats of physical harm: bank managers who rob their own bank because a gun is being held to their head. Such examples seem to have no parallel in health care. Whoever heard of patients being forced to have operations whilst at gunpoint? It is, however, a mistake to think of coercion only in these terms. Coercion can be unsubtle without being violent and can be so subtle that it is hardly recognized as such.

Fairly unsubtle coercion is one where a desired intervention is offered on condition that an undesired intervention is also accepted: for example, a termination of pregnancy is given only if the woman also agrees to a concurrent sterilization. Another fairly unsubtle way of coercing patients is the threat of withdrawing a desired intervention unless agreement to a further intervention is given. It is not, however, always the case that where one therapy is made dependent upon another that coercion has occurred but the line is a fine one. The difference depends upon the extent to which clinical judgement must be respected; the line is drawn at the point where clinical judgement becomes personal preference, prejudice, or ignorance.

On one level, it is obvious that clinical judgement has to be respected. Practitioners ought not to be forced to compromise or prostitute their skills and judgement to whim, but how is whim to be determined in this context? The case of home births illustrates the difficulties of both respecting professional judgement and allowing voluntary choice. Many obstetricians feel uncomfortable about agreeing to deliver babies at home. In some cases they will simply refuse to do so without any discussion or explanation and also refuse to cooperate with the patient's search for an alternative obstetrician. In other cases they tell the patient that, in their view, a home delivery will be so dangerous that they cannot be party to the risk and will not therefore attend the delivery. The extent to which such coercion is ethical depends, in part, upon the extent to which the home birth will be risky. If the risk lies in the particular woman's obstetric history, then the refusal might be more justified than if the objection is based on the view that all deliveries are risky until proven otherwise: in the latter case, the refusal seems less obviously one of clinical judgement. It is not clear that all deliveries are risky nor that these risks are more likely to manifest themselves in a home delivery. Refusal might also reflect the competing interests of other patients, which require the consultant to remain nearer to the hospital delivery suite, but this reflects the tensions of conflicting duties and utility rather than an ethical stand for clinical judgement as such. Not unreasonably, a consultant might also point out that if her attendance is deemed necessary, then the delivery is probably perceived as being a high-risk one anyway, and not, therefore advisable.

All practitioners should be free to *express* clinical judgement. It is not wrong for a practitioner to tell a patient that, in her opinion, a desired course of action is dangerous and to explain why this is so. It seems coercive, however, to withdraw all support unless agreement is reached. Equally, whilst it is easy to argue in favour of negotiation (for instance, to ask the woman what it is about a home delivery that cannot be provided by a hospital delivery and to try to accommodate these aspects within the hospital delivery), there will, from time to time, be patients who, for one reason or another, will not meet in the middle ground (and undoubtedly, there are professionals like this too!), in which case not to attend, for instance, a woman nearing the second stage of labour at home, in order to protect professional judgement would be unethical.

Subtle coercion occurs more indirectly often through verbal and non-verbal signals to the patient; examples include: treating a non-compliant patient more brusquely than other patients; emphasizing one therapy enthusiastically, whilst mentioning genuine alternatives only in passing; confusing the patient with jargon or overloading her with information (see Chapter 3). In midwifery, perhaps the most effective form of subtle coercion is the suggestion, in the face of resistance, that harm might come to the baby if advice is ignored. Tone of voice, tuts and hums can all be used to good effect to undermine a patient's confidence in her decision. Even here, though, there is a difference between coercion and expressing an opinion as such, or indeed making a recommendation in an environment where it is possible for this recommendation to be rejected. The duty to inform readily accommodates the expression of clinical judgement provided that, where appropriate, the practitioner makes clear the extent to which the verdict is an expression of her individual professional opinion rather than the consensus view of her profession.

Information

Being informed is one aspect of acting in a way that is voluntary. This mutual dependence is most vividly exemplified where the patient is intentionally deceived. If a patient acts in ignorance of the truth, then it is difficult to see how this decision can be described as voluntary. This is pretty clearcut. Less obvious is the amount of information that a patient requires to make a decision, especially as too much information can paralyse a patient into indecision and anxiety, an excuse readily offered by those who prefer to make decisions for their patients. As with much in health care ethics, the amount of information needed to make a decision is a matter of judgement and balance. The minimum would be to discuss options, risks and side-effects in the context of some diagnosis and prognosis, in a jargon-free style, offering an opportunity for questions and including an assessment at the level of the patient's understanding.

However, it is unrealistic to suggest that the patient should be informed of every possible alternative therapy and each and every side-effect or risk. What she requires is enough relevant information to make a considered judgement.

The required level of information is often discussed by academic lawyers since, if it can be shown that a patient was not properly informed, consent becomes invalidated and the relevant practitioner may face a tort for negligence or even battery. (In law, an act of battery is a contact with someone without their permission, be this any kind of touching or major surgery, the taking of blood or the giving of a bedbath.) There is, however, no legal consensus on the amount of information that a patient has to receive to give valid consent to a procedure (for a more detailed review see Braizier, 1992). Here, I refer to the law only to borrow some frameworks in which to discuss ethical aspects of giving information.

In law, it is vital that the patient at least understands the general nature of a procedure; for instance, no patient can consent to a sterilization without realizing that this means that they will no longer be able to have children. Apart from emergencies, the same applies to any woman consenting to a hysterectomy. Beyond this barest minimum, various suggestions about the amount of information needed have been made. In the UK, doctors are only required to give patients the information that is normally given to similar patients by their peers. 'Standard clinical practice', as this is called, only requires a doctor to show that a substantial body of his or her profession would have done the same thing to mount an effective defence against battery. This substantial body of opinion need only be a couple of expert witnesses, even if witnesses to the contrary are offered by the patient. Doctors are, however, obliged to answer a patient's questions honestly (unless it is not standard clinical practice to do so). This formula leaves the onus upon the patient to probe further if she is dissatisfied with the level of information given, which is difficult if she is unaware of which pertinent questions she should ask.

In the USA, the 'prudent patient' test is applied. Doctors are obliged to tell the patient anything that a prudent patient would want to know; but it is not always clear what is meaningful and useful to all patients.

One question that practitioners might usefully ask themselves is, 'Am I deliberately not mentioning something or deliberately emphasizing something in order to manipulate the patient into making a particular decision?' Or, 'How certain am I that this patient really knows what is going on?' A negative answer to this latter question may relate to things that the patient does not know; it may equally reflect the fact that the patient has become incapable of knowing what is going on, that she is now unable to understand the information being given.

Competence

The starting point for consent is actually competence. It is because one is competent to make the decision for oneself that one should be sufficiently informed and then permitted to make the choice. Competence is the foundation for autonomy, for whilst someone who is potentially autonomous can be deceived and misinformed, or someone who is potentially autonomous can be coerced to do something against her will, someone who is intrinsically or temporarily incompetent cannot be autonomous. A distinction must also be drawn between being incompetent and being irrational. Autonomous beings can take huge risks autonomously, provided that they understand the nature of those risks. Indeed, it is the ability to understand the nature of the risk which is central, rather than their ability to persuade a third party of the merits of risk-taking. There is a significant difference between accepting that someone is competent and agreeing with the decisions that they make for themselves. Unfortunately, some practitioners generate a faulty kind of syllogism to overcome this difference, which runs something like this:

> I am the expert in this field: you would be crazy to ignore my advice.
> You have ignored my advice, therefore you are crazy.
> You are crazy, therefore you are incompetent to make decisions for yourself.
> I am therefore justified in ignoring your incompetent wishes.

Competence is not an absolute state, though incompetence might be. Generally one's competence is relative to that which one is being asked to do. The patient's view regarding the practitioner may be, 'You are competent to deliver a baby, I am not, but this does not mean that as your patient I am incapable of consenting to the way in which my delivery is managed'. In the context of consent, competence means that one understands that one is being required to make a decision about oneself and also the information upon which this decision has to be based. Effectively, one also has to be in a position to express the result of this decision since if one is competent but unable (perhaps due to paralysis) to communicate, for the practical purposes of those trying to gain consent, one is rendered incompetent. Likewise, one might be competent to understand the relevant information but may be rendered incompetent by the ineffective communication skills of the practitioner attempting to give this information. It might also be that one is competent to form some kinds of judgement but not others because they are essentially more complex. This is not an observation unique to health care. It has been suggested on many occasions that ordinary jurors, for instance, are simply unable to grasp the complexities of some fraud cases and that they are therefore incompetent to make a judgement about the guilt or innocence of the defendant.

There is a tendency in health care to define certain *groups* of individuals as being incompetent. This should be resisted in most cases since it fails to account for the range of abilities within any group and also it fails to recognize that individuals are rarely incompetent *per se*. Rather they will be competent to make some decisions but not others. It is now being recognized, for instance, that children should not be assumed to be incompetent, though infants and babies may be. Likewise that the mentally disabled and ill are capable of consenting to some things, even quite complex things, if these are explained skilfully enough. However, it is clear that those who are unconscious are unable, for the time being at least, to make any of their own decisions.

For midwives, this general tendency to indentify groups of incompetent patients has been particularly fraught with ethical danger since one such group to be defined as incompetent has been women in labour. This is both because it is a painful process and because some of the drugs given to relieve pain may result in the patient becoming confused. Against this, it can be argued quite obviously, that labour comes in various stages, the pain varies from woman to woman and some forms of pain relief interfere with judgement less than others. So, while some women may become incompetent during periods of their confinement, not all women are incompetent through the whole process of childbirth. In addition, it is not uncommon in midwifery for women to make birth plans prior to their confinements, in effect consenting or refusing consent, in writing, prior to the event.

These 'advance directives' can generate problems if the woman changes her mind during the labour, especially if she has told her birth attendant and/or accompanying friend to disregard anything she says in contradiction of her birth plan once labour is underway.

As Rosalind Ekman Ladd points out, however, some of the consent forms (particularly in the USA) that women sign are not like other consent forms, living wills or advance directives because labouring women do not have the same 'escape hatches' as other patients (Ladd, 1992). If one signs a consent form prior to elective surgery, one can always discharge oneself from the hospital prior to being given the pre-medication; if one consents to be involved in clinical research, one can withdraw at any time from the trial. Moreover, she says, if one signs an advance directive, one can always rip it up if one changes one's mind; it does not come into force until one is incompetent. I agree with Ladd that since labour is an unavoidable and inevitable outcome of pregnancy one cannot just decide not to go through with the birth after all and leave the hospital. I also accept that in the USA, where signing an all-encompassing consent form may be a prerequisite to being accepted into the care of a hospital consultant, many women have little choice but to sign and little room for manoeuvre having signed. However, in the UK I do not think that the birth plan drawn up with the midwife is, or should be, granted absolute status. As with an advance directive, the woman can change her mind at any time before labour and expect her new wishes to be given equal respect. I do grant though, that labouring women are in a more difficult position because of the general tendency to assume that labouring women are in too much pain and too afraid to make competent decisions. I also grant that some women may be in agony when they change their mind about an epidural, but what an excellent and completely understandable reason to change one's mind! I likewise think that if someone in such pain is able to continue to refuse an epidural then, because they are refusing in the light of such pain, this is a good reason to respect their sincerity. It is unreasonable of pregnant women or their attendants to try to agree upon precisely how a delivery will be managed down to the last injection or whiff of gas, when each delivery is different and until it is happening it is not possible to predict how it will feel; there are too many variables.

Possibly, part of the problem of consent in this context is that too much emphasis is placed on making contracts prior to the event and too little on women being able to consent whilst in labour. In this respect, there is a huge difference between expressing a preference and actually contracting to do something. Whilst I might agree with my friend that, for her, a birth without pain relief seems desirable, I would not agree forcibly to prevent anyone giving her pain relief if she found that she could not bear it at the time. The process of gaining consent prior to labour should be a process of counselling and an exchange of information, rather than a contract. The aim should be to facilitate discussion of what can reasonably be expected to happen under a variety of circumstances.

This process of understanding and negotiation should be, and probably is, the norm in modern midwifery practice. There will, however, be occasions when a woman will absolutely insist on a contract kind of refusal of consent; for instance, refusal of a blood transfusion if she is a Jehovah's Witness. I will deal with such cases later as ones of conflict of interests rather than a problem with competence as such, since it is already well established that a patient who refuses such therapy when competent cannot be given it when she is no longer competent simply because she is now unable to object.

Decision

There is a difference between making a decision and acquiescing. Decision-making is a conscious process, whereas to acquiesce is to agree without reflection. Acquiescing is also different to the conscious decision to allow another to make the decision. Making a decision is the final stage in the process of giving consent. It is also the final point in the process of refusing consent. A valid refusal of consent should be as binding as valid consent. Understandably, when a patient refuses to do something that her carer thinks is in her best interests, her decision is more likely to be questioned than if consent is forthcoming. However, this does not make obvious sense, for if the patient was competent to consent, then she was equally competent to refuse consent. If the carer was happy to give a procedure on the grounds that consent was received, she should be equally comfortable accepting that the procedure cannot now go ahead, unless, of course, it can be shown that a greater degree of competence is required to oppose professional recommendation than to accept it. Many practitioners seem happy to perform procedures provided their patients simply acquiesce, but this is not obvious until a situation arises where a similar patient refuses to consent.

An argument can be made for applying stricter criteria to refusal in the face of definite advice, provided that it can be shown that the refusal fundamentally alters the gravity of the decision. This is an argument which is applied particularly when a patient is refusing a life-saving therapy. Buchanan and Brock (1989) suggest that the greater the risks being taken, the greater the need to examine the capacity for competent decision making. This, they claim, accords not only with the law but also common sense. We would, for instance, be prepared to let a child determine what they ate for lunch, but not whether and where to invest huge sums of money (Buchanan and Brock, 1989). It is not, however, clear why it is risk *per se* which makes all the difference rather than simply the complexity of the decision required. This point is made by Wicclair (1991) when he modifies the lunch example by asking us to suppose that the child's choice will actually produce a violent allergic reaction in that child. It is not the risk of the violent reaction that renders the child unable to choose, but rather doubts about whether the child understands what a violent allergic reaction is. If the child does not understand, then it is not a matter of being paternalistic when choosing their lunch but rather it is a case of making a proxy decision (Wicclair, 1991).

Thus, when determining the validity of a patient's refusal of consent, a minimum *competence* test (which varies according to the complexity of the decision) provides greater protection to patient autonomy than a minimum *risk* test, though the latter may provide better protection from harm for the patient as perceived by others.

Paternalism and proxy decisions

Paternalism occurs when someone's *capacity* to make their own decision is ignored. It can take the form of overriding an actual decision, not bothering to get a decision in the first place, or deliberately manipulating a decision by misleading the patient through the information given or withheld. Employing any of these techniques invalidates consent and renders the procedure concerned *involuntary*. A clear distinction needs to be kept between involuntary and *non-voluntary* which refers to action taken without the patient's consent because the patient is incompetent to consent. Paternalism occurs when a procedure is carried out involuntarily. Where an action is non-voluntary it results from a *proxy* or *surrogate* decision.

Paternalism and proxy decision making are easily confused because, however misguided, paternalism is essentially benevolent. Someone acting paternalistically is motivated by the desire to do the best for the subject of their attention, just like those who make proxy decisions. The difference is that whereas the subject of the proxy decision is incapable of making a choice, the paternalist considers that they know better than the subject where the subject's best interests lie. So, to perform an episiotomy against a woman's wishes because one envisages extensive tearing is paternalistic. To decide to perform an episiotomy whilst the woman is delirious (and thereby incompetent) from pain and analgesics is to make a proxy decision. These distinctions can be made without judging either to be the correct or the wrong response. The road to hell may be paved with good intentions, but even so there is a significant difference between actions that are motivated by benevolence and those that are performed indifferently or even maliciously.

There is considerable debate over who is best placed to act as proxy, particularly for small children. In the labour suite, the same kind of debate may occur between the doctor, midwife and accompanying friend of the patient, each of whom can make a strong case for being the one to decide on an incompetent patient's behalf. One difference between children and pregnant women in this regard is that pregnant women can actually specify in advance whose judgement they wish to take precedence. Practitioners are unlikely to find this a problem when it is they whom the patient designates. On the other hand, if it is the friend, hostility can be generated. Nevertheless, in ethical terms, provided that the patient specified that the friend act as the proxy, then if the patient's autonomy must be respected so should the decisions of her designated proxy.

It is possible that the attempt to reject the patient's appointed proxy by the professional carer is an indication of a deeper problem than simply that of determining who is in the best position to decide on the patient's behalf. Anyone's commitment to the principle of respecting autonomy would be severely tested under circumstances where the patient is slowly dying because the proxy is refusing some procedure like a blood transfusion. Refusing to acknowledge the status of a proxy enables carers to avoid the issue of the extent to which we are free to make decisions that might result in our being seriously harmed. This leads us to a series of specific questions about the limits that can be legitimately placed upon a patient's autonomy.

Limits to autonomy

Can a woman bring harm on herself?

In order to avoid repeating material covered above in this section, the specific question of whether one can autonomously harm oneself, and if so, under what circumstances will be discussed.

It is clear that our autonomous choices are not restricted to acting only in our own interests, at least not if these are narrowly defined. We frequently do things which we might otherwise not do when asked by someone we love. We devote more time to work than we are strictly paid to do, when someone needs us, or to help out a colleague. Many parents would willingly sacrifice their lives to save those of their children. Such examples illustrate the sense in which we autonomously choose to limit our actions in ways that do not apparently directly advantage us. Clearly, it could be argued that really we are not harmed by so doing because it serves our longer term interests in some kind of you-scratch-my-back-I'll-scratch-yours social contract sense. But what about the decision to die for our children? Here it is not so clear that our long-term interests are served, since we will no longer be around to reap the benefits.

In this case, it is not that our wider interests are served, but rather that there are at least some things that we value more than ourselves: the lives of our children perhaps. There are other things that people have been willing to die for too: their religious amd political beliefs, for example. In such cases, even though we do not necessarily share the views of those willing to make the sacrifice, we often do accept that they should be free to make such choices and we do not always find such decisions to be irrational. The extent to which we find such decisions to be irrational depends, in large measure, on whether we think that the end of the action is actually something inherently more valuable than life.

It seems, then, that a substantial part of our willingness to accept the self-harming actions of patients will flow from the coherence to us of the justification that they give for their actions. The danger of using this as the sole basis of determining whether or not patients should be free to make their own decisions, is that it is an invitation for unlimited paternalism, with patients only being given the freedom to choose what would, in any case, have been chosen for them. We must be in a position to determine whether the difference of judgement here turns on some kind of faulty decision-making capacity of the patient or whether the disagreement is essentially one between different values. For this reason, we need a fairly rigorous but tolerant notion of what constitutes a coherent justification.

One aspect of a coherent justification for an action would be to consider whether or not the decision was consistent with the values the patient claimed to hold: to ask, does it facilitate the state of affairs that the patient desires, or hinder it? In this sense, the decision being made could be said to reflect the patient's true self.

Even if one is assured that the patient's decision-making faculty is not impaired, one might still wonder whether the decision has been made autonomously, for one might question whether the values that underpin the decision were actually autonomously chosen. Many of our values reflect social conditioning, family influence and so forth and do not result from considered reflection. However, since this is true of so many of us, is it reasonable to expect patients refusing intervention to be better able to justify the values that they hold than other people, or indeed patients complying with treatment recommendations? Equally, it is also necessary to recognize instances where there is more reason to question the autonomous decision to hold one set of values rather than another.

One such case was tested in court. A pregnant woman was admitted to hospital accompanied by her mother, who was a Jehovah's Witness. The daughter had been raised by her father, who was not a Witness, after her mother left home. At the time of admission to hospital, there was no reason to suppose that a blood transfusion would be necessary. However, after being alone for several hours with her mother, the daughter mentioned to the nurse that she would not wish to be given a blood transfusion should it become necessary to have one. Unfortunately, following the birth of a stillborn baby by Caesarean section, a transfusion was indicated but the staff were reluctant to give one since the daughter was both an adult and had appeared competent at the time her instruction was issued. Her father was incensed, convinced that the mother had taken the opportunity to brainwash their daughter whilst she was vulnerable and susceptible to persuasion. He successfully petitioned for the blood to be given. Here the issue was not one of whether religious views should be accepted, whatever the consequences for the believer, but rather whether the supposed believer freely held the religious views she used to justify her decision (*Re T*, 1992).

Examples such as this one are exceptional. Less exceptional, but still rare, are cases where women refuse to have a Caesarean section because they find the prospect terrifying. Here again, the decision-making faculty might not be impaired, but terror of surgery might be difficult to accept as a valid reason to refuse it. In these, and other exceptional cases, the best that one can do is tread the fine line between genuinely attempting to respect autonomy and also genuinely attempting to ascertain just how voluntary the decision in question is. The role of the professional carer is perhaps more clearcut, where the decision in question affects not just the mother, but also the fetus.

Can a woman make decisions, the effects of which bring harm to the fetus?

I am deliberately going to limit my discussions here to the actions of women who intend to take their pregnancies to term. Excluded, then, is the decision to have a termination of pregnancy, which is clearly the most common decision made by women that could be said to harm the fetus.

It is generally held that whilst we are free to bring harm upon ourselves, we are not free to bring harm upon others. However, this is not an absolute rule, since it is applied under a presumption in favour of autonomy. This means that some harm to others is tolerated where this harm is minor and the cost of preventing it, in terms of individual liberty, would be great. Our autonomy would be virtually worthless if this were not so, since almost any action we take has harmful side-effects on someone. Travelling by train might be less damaging to the environment, but that does not mean that no damage to the environment is caused by trains. However, the more serious the harm, the more likely we are to allow the sacrifice of individual freedom to avoid it.

The difficulty with applying this general principle in the case of pregnant women is that in attempting to resolve the competing interests, the fetus's interest in not being harmed and the woman's interest in her autonomy, we recognize that avoiding harm to the fetus can require much more of an imposition on the woman than avoiding harm generally requires. It may require an actual bodily intrusion, like a Caesarean section, keyhole surgery or the taking of some drug. At the other end of the spectrum, it might entail some behaviour modification by the patient, and somewhere in the middle, interference with her views about the mode of her confinement, which may, under some circumstances, compromise her ideals.

One way of analysing this problem is to see it as a conflict between maternal and fetal rights: the woman's rights over her own body versus the fetus's right not to be harmed. Into this conflict, people then bring their views about the status of the fetus (either comparing the fetus to any other person and awarding strong claims in terms of their interests, or holding that the fetus has no claims, either due to gestational development or due to dependence upon and location within the mother's body). Also, they bring their views about the obligations of the pregnant woman, some holding that women who are pregnant have special obligations to their fetus by virtue of choosing to go ahead with the pregnancy, or that the obligations are no different to those that could be expected of any other person whose liberty was being curtailed to a similar degree.

There is not space here to extend this rather intractable debate. My own position is that at least *some* pregnant women do have special obligations to their fetus(es), but this is not by virtue of having chosen to continue with the pregnancy *per se*, but by virtue of having taken on the mantle of motherhood (which is not something all pregnant women have done; an obvious example here would be a woman acting as a surrogate or one who has decided to offer the baby for adoption).

The possibilities afforded by modern technology have resulted in debate about the true nature of motherhood, posing questions such as whether motherhood is based on genetic relationships, bearing a baby or rearing a child. Perhaps motherhood can more accurately be defined in terms of a moral relationship, where a woman takes on certain moral obligations towards a particular child. If this is so, then the very least that such an obligation would entail is that of care and nurture. In this case, a mother might be obliged to accept more of an infringement of her liberties for the protection of her child than another person might be expected to endure for the protection of someone else's child. This does not mean that pregnant mothers are obliged to do anything, no matter how serious the consequences for themselves, for the benefit of the fetus. Instead, it means that mothers would be obliged to undertake major infringements of liberty where it could be shown that this would definitely be of major benefit to the fetus. The less definite the benefit, or the less the benefit, the less sacrifice mothers are obliged to make, though a minor sacrifice for a small benefit would also be acceptable. Women who have chosen to continue with a pregnancy for reasons other than to be mothers do have obligations to consider the interests of the future child, but this is not a special obligation, rather it is on a par with the obligations generally placed on any of us not to cause unnecessary harm. Such a general obligation may require significantly less self-sacrifice than that placed on mothers, or so it could be argued.

Here, I am relying on mothers to moderate their own behaviour according to their own beliefs about what is in the best interests of their child. Quite a different set of arguments would be needed to compel mothers to make these sacrifices. The very least such a justification would require is that either all parents (both fathers and mothers) be prepared so to sacrifice, or that all people would be prepared so to sacrifice, even for strangers. This is a view that I have developed elsewhere (Draper, 1996).

Conclusion

An argument that does not permit midwives to impose a therapy upon a pregnant women, even though the failure to do so will result in enormous harm to the fetus, might seem useless to those in the field. Perhaps the lesson to be learned from this is that there is an ethical, and as well as pragmatic, need to negotiate with pregnant women before emergencies arise. If it is the case that women enter into pregnancies with certain expectations about the care that they will receive and also presuming that nothing will go wrong for them, this is, perhaps, the fault of the health care professionals who have, in the past, promised more than they are able to deliver. If labouring women are distrustful of the advice that they are given, this is perhaps because so many procedures have, previously, been given for spurious clinical reasons or for the convenience of carers. Just as there are good grounds for arguing that mothers have to take their ethical responsibilities for their fetuses seriously, professionals can also be charged with obligations to ensure that the information they give to women as part of gaining consent is true, based in sound research and up-to-date.

References

Brazier, M. (1992). *Medicine, Patients and the Law.* Penguin Books.
Buchanan, A. E. and Brock, D. W. (1989). *Deciding for Others.* Cambridge University Press.
Culver, C. and Gert, B. (1982). *Philosophy and Medicine.* Oxford University Press.
Draper, H. (forthcoming). Women, forced caesarean and antenatal responsibilities. *J. Med. Ethics* (in press).
Gillon, R. (1986). *Philosophical Medical Ethics.* John Wiley.
Ladd, R. E. (1992). Women in labour: some issues in informed consent. In *Feminist Perspectives in Medical Ethics* (H. B. Holmes and L. M. Purdy, eds) pp. 216–223. Indiana University Press.
Re, T. (1992). 4 *All England Law Reports*, p. 649.
Scoccia, D. (1990). Paternalism and respect for autonomy. *Ethics*, 100, 2.
Wicclair, M. R. (1991). Patient decision making: Capacity and risk. *Bioethics*, 15 (2), 118–122.

Chapter 2

Choices in childbirth: Areas of conflict

Helen Lewison

Introduction

There has been an increase in the academic consideration of midwifery ethics, but how is ethics working in practice at the grass roots level in the interactions between the ordinary woman and the ordinary midwife? There is no doubt that a growth in literature particular to the ethics of midwifery is to be welcomed as further evidence that midwifery is a separate profession. However, ethics in childbirth is rarely considered from the point of view of the woman. This chapter therefore attempts to redress the balance by exploring the ethical issues from the woman's point of view and also from outside the profession, since the author is neither a midwife nor an ethicist, but works as a user representative for maternity services.

The legal and ethical framework within which conflicts of choice occur

The midwifery profession is governed by a detailed framework of both primary and secondary legislation that is intended to protect the public. This legislation is the product of the Judaeo–Christian framework that regulates British society despite the many cultures and religions espoused by the people of our increasingly diverse society. The area within this framework is where ethics or the 'rules of conduct' (*Concise Oxford Dictionary*, 1990) operate and are employed by all those concerned with maternity services. These include:

- women and their families;
- midwives;
- doctors;
- other caregivers;
- employees and non-executive members of NHS trusts;
- employees and non-executive members of district health authorities and regional offices;
- employees and members of community health councils;
- employees and volunteer workers of the maternity user organizations such as the National Childbirth Trust;
- employees of the Department of Health, including the NHS Executive.

All the above individuals and organizations are stakeholders in maternity services and thus bring their own ethical perspectives to bear on individual recipients of care, on elements of the system as well as the system as a whole. In practice, all these perspectives operate as constantly shifting constructs of overlapping and interweaving interests nudging, overlaying and influencing each other.

Informed choice

Informed choice is now seen as the fundamental right of every woman having a baby if she is to retain her autonomy in childbearing (Department of Health, 1993). Modern medicine is experiencing a shift from paternalism grounded in beneficence to increasing service user autonomy, thus giving the woman responsibility for her own decisions.

Informed choice must be distinguished from consent. Consent is important from the midwife's point of view, as it is the bare minimum required by law to authorize any procedure carried out by the midwife. Whilst verbal consent has the same legal force as written consent, it is, of course, much harder to substantiate after the event. Informed choice is more important from the woman's point of view as it reflects a genuine understanding of the issues. This is particularly important when there is no evidence to show that in terms of anticipated outcome, one choice is not as good as another. Therefore, from a pragmatic as well as an ethical point of view, this decision might as well be made by the woman. The Winterton Report (Health Select Committee, 1992) stated:

> We conclude that until such time as there is more detailed and accurate research about such interventions as epidurals, episiotomies, caesarean sections, electronic fetal monitoring, instrumental delivery and induction of labour, women need to be given a choice on the basis of existing information rather than having to undergo such interventions as routine.

The International Code of Ethics for Midwives has as the first article of its code: 'Midwives must respect a woman's informed right of choice and promote the woman's acceptance of responsibility for the outcomes of her choices' (International and Confederation of Midwives, 1993). It defines 'informed' in this context as implying: 'that complete information is given to and understood by the woman regarding the risks, benefits and probable outcomes of each choice available to her'.

This is a high standard to be achieved in an area of health care where choices can be complex. In addition, historically in the health services as a whole, health professionals have been reluctant to share either information or decision-making with their clients. This is in marked contrast to the attitude of, for example, the legal professions where great pains have always been taken to explain to clients the possible options for action and the likely outcomes of any choice. Government-led initiatives such as the Patient's Charter (Department of Health, 1995) and the Patient's Charter for Maternity Services (Department of Health, 1994) are beginning to raise basic standards. However, this is a long way from empowering every user of the health service to be able to make informed choices.

Two obstacles stand in the way of women becoming empowered and hence able to make informed choices: the low information base with which the majority of women embark on pregnancy and, in some cases, an alleged reluctance to take responsibility for making difficult choices in pregnancy and labour. This failure to take responsibility is usually anecdotal and not based on formal evidence. In contrast, what little research there is shows a willingness by women to make informed choices (Green et al., 1990), but a reluctance on

the part of midwives to give women sufficient information on which
to base informed decisions (Kirkham, 1989).

Some well-educated women enthusiastically read everything they
can lay their hands on so they can make informed choices. For others
this is more difficult, either for socio-economic reasons or because
they do not read or understand English. For women brought up in
other countries, it is hard enough to understand the system, let alone
make complex choices about antenatal screening or pain relief in
labour. This is an area where the midwife can choose to educate the
woman herself. This can be done, for example, by learning the
language of the local ethnic minority community or by ensuring that
an interpreter is present at every antenatal consultation. Alternatively,
she can facilitate learning by the woman in other ways, such as
referring her to special classes held in her own community or by
lending her audio-cassette tapes and videos in her own language. This
can be difficult if the necessary resources are not available at local
level. In such cases, the midwife's effectiveness in promoting informed
choice is limited by circumstances. However, the International Code
of Ethics (International Confederation of Midwives, 1993) states:
'Midwives, together with women, should work with policy and
funding agencies to define women's needs for health services and to
ensure that resources are fairly allocated considering priorities and
availability'. From this it is clear that the midwife, both as a partner
and an advocate for women, should be working at the appropriate
level open to her, be it local, regional or national, to secure resources
in order that more women can achieve such informed decision-making.
At the local level, the district health authority has a duty to assess
and provide for the needs of the local population. The Maternity
Services Liaison Committee (MSLC), if properly constituted (Lewison,
1994), should have midwifery representation and, in its role as an
advisory group to the district health authority, be working towards
making maternity services woman centred and conducive to the
making of informed choices by women at every stage of their care.

Facilitating informed choice is likely to become a more important
dimension in the role of all midwives and this should form a major
part of each consultation between a woman and her midwife. All
such discussions and the choices made should be written in the
maternity record. It will often be relevant and helpful to record the
reasons for any advice given and the basis on which women have
made their choices. It is felt by some midwives that such careful

record-keeping is part of a defensive approach to care and is out of keeping with the traditional role of the midwife. Others feel that it is an integral part of a high standard of midwifery care (Symon, 1994). Rule 42(1) of the Midwives Rules provides that: 'A practising midwife shall keep as contemporaneously as is reasonable detailed records of observations, care given and medicine or other forms of pain relief administered to all mothers and babies' (UKCC, 1993).

It could be argued that the meaning of 'care' in the above context includes information-giving, discussions and decision-making, particularly in view of the first of the three key principles of *Changing Childbirth* which states: 'The woman must be the focus of maternity care. She should be able to feel that she is in control of what is happening to her and able to make decisions about her care, based on her needs, having discussed matters fully with the professionals involved' (Department of Health, 1993).

Now that the implementation of the recommendations of *Changing Childbirth* has become government policy (NHS Management Executive, 1994), it seems fair that decisions by both the woman and the midwife and the reasons for them should be recorded. The first indicator of the success of *Changing Childbirth* is that, 'All women should be entitled to carry their own notes' (Department of Health, 1993). As larger numbers of women carry their own maternity record (Fawdry, 1994) and even fill in parts of their notes for themselves (Galloway, 1994), they should become able to understand more fully the reasons for different procedures and the advice given. In this way they are likely to be more involved in decision-making throughout pregnancy, labour and postnatally.

As women become more experienced in making informed choices about such issues as place of birth, style of antenatal care and antenatal screening, they may become more able and willing to make informed choices about interventions in labour. These might include routine artificial rupture of the membranes on admission into hospital in early labour; the method of fetal heart rate monitoring in uncomplicated labour; and the position for delivery: all decisions which historically have been made by midwives on their behalf (Garcia and Garforth, 1989).

Some women may choose to be guided by the advice of their caregivers in the case of complications, for example whether an assisted delivery should be performed using Ventouse or forceps. When there are problems in a pregnancy, this inevitably leads to a reduction in some choices but there may be other choices to be made. For instance, the birth may be safer in hospital and, if a Caesarean section is necessary, a choice of general or regional anaesthesia may be offered. In all these cases, however, it is possible to convey the reasons for an intervention being necessary and for one option being recommended in preference to another. Even in an emergency there is time for information to be conveyed sensitively and informed consent to be sought. The midwife present, particularly if she has spent some time with the woman during labour, is ideally placed to answer questions and to check that the woman has understood what is happening and why.

Choice is meaningless unless it is a real choice between two viable alternatives. Too often, women are forced into choosing between the lesser of two evils rather than choosing something they really want. For example, a woman may choose a home birth in order to receive care from one or two midwives because there is no Domino or similar integrated midwifery scheme providing continuity of carer for women preferring to give birth in hospital. In a similar way, some women who wish for a Domino-type birth when the quota is full circumvent the system by asking for a home birth, whereupon they are suddenly offered a package of care of this kind.

Whilst every maternity service will have some constraints on offering all possible choices, consideration should be given to providing the widest range of choice possible. For example, it will be necessary when induction of labour takes place for a woman who has booked a home birth to be admitted into hospital. The woman's disappointment might be mitigated if she could be admitted into hospital on the morning of the day chosen for the procedure and be attended by the community midwives whom she knows, rather than to be admitted the night before, undergo a separation from her partner at a stressful time and be attended by hospital midwives whom she does not know (of course, a system of integrated midwifery care dispenses with this problem).

Where do conflicts of choice occur?

Conflicts of choice can occur at every level in the system and between any combination of stakeholders, including a woman and the midwife caring for her. One example of this might be a situation where a woman is in labour in hospital and her preferred way of coping with the pain of labour is to have the constant physical and emotional support of a midwife. This might not be possible for a number of reasons.

- The midwife does not believe that this kind of support is effective. Here the conflict arises from the midwife's ignorance of research findings such as those collected in the Cochrane Pregnancy and Childbirth Database.
- The midwife does not believe that this support will be effective for this woman, because she looks like the sort of woman who needs an epidural, although her labour is uncomplicated. Here, the midwife is refusing to respect the woman's autonomy to make her own choices and to change her mind, if she wishes, in her own time.
- The midwife does not like giving this support and finds an excuse not to do so. Here it could be argued that a midwife is refusing to give support which could reasonably be expected by a woman from a midwife.
- The midwife, unbidden, gives the woman an injection of pethidine, saying, 'This will help you relax and make the pain easier to bear.' Here, the midwife has infringed the woman's autonomy by not seeking her informed consent.
- The midwife is unable to give this support because she is looking after several women in labour at the same time, a regular occurrence in many hospitals. Here, the woman's choice is in conflict with the hospital's preferred deployment of resources.

Another example of a situation where conflict can occur is if a labour ward protocol is inconsistent with research findings. It might provide, for example, that all women when admitted into hospital in labour should have their membranes broken artificially as a matter of routine, even when there is no clinical indication to do so. A woman might have learned from her reading or from antenatal classes that in an uncomplicated labour nothing is gained from routine artificial rupture of the membranes and, on the contrary, she is likely to find contractions more painful than if the membranes were left intact. Here, the conflict arises from routine protocols not being based on evidence.

While the ultimate aim of this chapter is to promote awareness of areas of conflict in everyday practice, it is helpful to consider the East

Herts water birth case. Although it is rather an unusual and extreme case, and for that very reason captured the attention of the media at the time, it demonstrates several areas of conflict in high relief.

The East Herts water birth case

The East Herts NHS Trust had a policy of allowing women to labour, but not to give birth in water. A mother had informed the two midwives with whom she had booked a home birth that she intended to labour at home in a hired birthing pool and that she wished to keep her options open about delivering in water.

The midwives, who had not delivered a baby in water before, asked permission for paid leave to observe some water births in hospitals elsewhere. This was refused. Therefore the midwives prepared themselves by reading the relevant literature and hiring a video showing a delivery under water. They then informed the woman that, as far as they could see, there was no inherent danger in a water delivery, provided the labour was uncomplicated. The woman was safely delivered of a baby daughter and was reported to have said afterwards that at the end of the second stage she would have found it very difficult to climb out of the pool to give birth.

However, disciplinary action was instigated against the midwives for breach of the Trust's protocol. One midwife received a final written warning which meant that she would be dismissed if she committed another transgression in the next two years. The other midwife received a 'first written warning' and was required to undergo three months' updating.

The UKCC supported the action of the midwives, maintaining that delivering babies in water is not a new 'treatment'. The Royal College of Midwives (RCM) sought judicial review on the basis that the actions of the Trust were not fair and equitable. The RCM also investigated with their solicitors whether there were grounds for civil action against the Trust for incitement to trespass. Both the RCM and the UKCC rapidly published documents on water birth to clarify the position of the midwife, which was to support the woman in her choice of a hitherto unevaluated practice (Royal College of Midwives, 1994; UKCC, 1994b). In addition, the midwives received the support of two user organizations, the National Childbirth Trust and the Association for Improvements in Maternity Services.

The practice of labouring in water was introduced into the UK in the 1980s by Dr Michel Odent. He recognized its value in helping women to relax and reduce the pain of labour, but did not at the time recommend it for delivery. However, some women preferred to stay in the pool for the birth and the midwives attending them learned how to manage delivery in this situation. It is estimated that in 1993 about 20 000 births took place with the help of water (Chapman, 1994) and that about 5% of women wish to have a water birth (Burns, 1993). An increasing number of hospitals have installed birthing pools in response to requests from women. There is, as yet, little systematic research into water births. The Department of Health has recognized the need for reliable evidence and is funding a study by the National Perinatal Epidemiology Unit into current practice. This had already begun at the time when water births received a burst of publicity in the media when a Swedish baby died in a water birth at home in 1993.

On examination these events reveal a complex web of conflicting issues and unresolved questions. On the face of it, the midwives were in breach of the protocol of the NHS Trust which required them to deliver the woman's baby on dry land. However, given the woman's refusal to leave the pool, they had only three choices when attending her in labour:

(1) to abandon the woman: this would have put them in breach of their statutory duty to attend her (Midwives Rules 40(1); UKCC, 1993);
(2) to manhandle her out of the water: this might have given rise to a charge of battery;
(3) to follow the woman's wishes and deliver the baby into water, which is what they did.

It is difficult to see what else the midwives could have done. Is the problem that both the woman and the midwives were open about her intentions? Should the midwives have tried harder to persuade the woman to deliver on dry land? Should the woman, as other women have done in different circumstances, have complied with the protocol antenatally and then only at the last minute have declared her intention to stay in the water to deliver her baby? Instead, the woman thought through the choices available to her and, both sensibly and considerately, communicated her wishes to her midwives antenatally.

Should the midwives have kept their counsel and not revealed the wishes of their client? Instead, the midwives, acting in accordance with their statutory duty (UKCC, 1994a), sought to update themselves on the management of water births. They also informed their supervisor of midwives who visited the woman at home antenatally.

Was the force of the protocol any different from any other protocol for the management of labour? In other situations, a woman can choose not to accept the requirements of a protocol. In these circumstances the woman's choice overrides the protocol since any intervention routinely proposed cannot be forced on her, provided that the discussion with her midwife or doctor is accurately recorded and that those attending her are not negligent, the woman takes responsibility for the outcome of her choice. Examples include a situation where a woman refuses artificial rupture of the membranes in an uncomplicated labour where the protocol provides that membranes should be ruptured routinely on admission into hospital; or where a woman exercises her pseudo-right to have her first baby at home, when the local criteria for home births exclude primigravidae (there is no statutory right to have a home birth: it is a pseudo-right because a woman cannot be forced to go to a hospital to have her baby).

Should the midwives have gone to court for an order to enforce the protocol on the woman? In the case of *Re S* (1992), a woman refused to accept medical advice to have her baby, which was lying in a transverse position, delivered by Caesarean section. A declaration was obtained to authorize the hospital staff to carry out an emergency Caesarean operation. Although the grounds for this decision were not explicit, it was thought that the order was granted to save the baby's life. The mother did not appeal against the declaration and in the event the baby died shortly before the Caesarean section was performed. There is some doubt in legal circles as to the validity of this decision, since the fetus has no rights in English law while *in utero*. In the case of the East Herts water birth, there was no evidence at any time that the baby's life was in danger, so it is unlikely that a court order would have been granted.

Did the Trust use research-based evidence to draft their protocol after the death of the Swedish baby? There is no evidence to show that it is less safe to deliver in water than on dry land, provided that the labour is uncomplicated and the baby is lifted out of the water immediately after birth. Where the evidence is unclear or insufficient to prevent or support a particular practice, is it not reasonable to accede to a woman's wishes and allow her to choose, rather than to impose a flawed blanket protocol? Both the Winterton Report (Health Select Committee, 1992) and *Changing Childbirth* (Department of Health, 1993) support the woman's right to choose in such circumstances. As shown above, even where there is evidence to support a particular practice, the woman's wishes have to be respected unless a court order can be obtained. It is unlikely that such an order would be granted without appropriate legislation being passed.

With hindsight, it is possible to analyse the conflict stemming from the fact that the East Herts NHS Trust protocol forbidding delivery in water was no more based on research than the woman's wish to keep open her options for delivering her baby into water. Was it therefore right for the Trust to discipline the two midwives for being in breach of a protocol based not on research but, apparently, drafted in reaction to the death of a baby in Sweden?

Why was it that midwives appeared to have been disciplined for supporting a woman's right to choose? It is possible that other problems lurk at a deeper level, such as a woman and her midwives working together to help her take control of her care (see Chapter 12).

It could be argued that the Trust's reaction to the woman asserting control over the manner of her birth was in some ways similar to that of the obstetrician who went to court in *Re S* (1992). It is possible that both the Trust and the obstetrician acted out of fear: the Trust afraid that they would be sued in the event of a baby dying during a water birth, the obstetrician that he would be held responsible if the baby died, despite attempts to persuade the woman to have a Caesarean section. These fears lacked any rational basis, since in both cases the appropriate steps had been taken to ensure that the women understood the implications of their decisions. Another interpretation is that the refusal of these women to, in one case, conform to the Trust's protocol, and in the other, to accept medical advice, were both interpreted as bids to exercise autonomy which heralded an unacceptable transfer of power to the hitherto powerless stakeholder in maternity care, the woman. By taking the action they did, it is as if both the Trust and the obstetrician were warning other women not to do the same.

A significant difference though, is that the Trust chose to take disciplinary action against two of its employees rather than attempt some form of action against the woman. The latter course was not open to them because the woman was within her rights, legally as well as morally, to give birth to her baby in water. What foundation, therefore, was there for the Trust's action against the midwives? Legally, although the midwives were in breach of the Trust's protocol, as has been shown above, they would have been in breach of their professional duty if they had followed any course of action other than the one they chose. Following orders is no defence against a breach of professional duty to one's client. Therefore there was no legal basis for the Trust's action. Morally it could be argued that the direct attempt to limit the midwives' professional autonomy was at the same time an indirect attempt to limit the autonomy of any woman wishing to deliver her baby in water in the future. Women generally tend to be protective of midwives; few women would be prepared to render their midwives vulnerable to disciplinary action if it could be avoided. Alternatively, was the Trust's action an attempt to save the lives of future babies? To regard a woman as merely a vessel for a fetus again fails to respect the autonomy of the woman. In addition, such a position is inconsistent with the moral climate of a society whose Abortion Act (1967) permits therapeutic abortion: is the moral status of a fetus at term superior to that of a fetus at 24 weeks? Thus, it can be argued that there was also no moral basis for the Trust's action.

It is significant that the UKCC's position statement (UKCC, 1994b) on water birth, published after the event, says:

> The Council recognises that employing authorities will wish to develop local policies in relation to the delivery of maternity services. In accordance with the Midwife's Code of Practice (paragraph 22) the Council considers it essential for supervisors of midwives and other practising midwives to be actively involved in the development of such policies. The purpose should be to ensure that these policies recognize fully the role and responsibilities of the midwife and, above all else, the woman's right to choose.

This gives rise to the further question: to what extent were the local midwives, including their supervisor, involved in the development of the East Herts NHS Trust protocol on water birth? The current trend in industry is increasingly to promote the autonomy of employees by encouraging them to participate in policy, planning and monitoring activities. The basis for this approach appears to be not only the utilitarian objective of a happier and more effective workforce, but also the rights-based principle that employees should be treated in as egalitarian way as is consistent with their abilities to contribute. If midwives were not involved with the formulation of the protocol, it is suggested that the Trust was out of step with the current climate of including employees in processes and enabling them to own the standards to which they have to work.

Conclusion: How can choice be extended and conflicts avoided?

Changing Childbirth (Department of Health, 1993) and its recommendations are based on the principle of autonomy, enabling the woman to exercise informed choice supported by health care givers who respect her autonomy and work in multidisciplinary teams in a manner which respects each other's professional autonomy. The fact that implementation of the report's recommendations is required by 1999 (NHS Management Executive, 1994) is likely to mean that women will increasingly be able to exercise more choice. At the same time, the report's focus on care becoming woman-centred and research-based should result in fewer conflicts of the kind described above.

However, during the interim period of transition, the following recommendations might make things easier for both women and midwives in the short term.

- To give women full, unbiased information in a form that can be understood by them, using alternative media and interpreters where necessary, as well as face to face contact.
- For midwives and other health professionals to learn that helping women to exercise autonomy and accept responsibility for their decisions is not only ethically acceptable but is also liberating for the health professional. Provided that the care giver has given the best care they can and ensured that the woman is informed of the full implications of her decision, they have fulfilled their moral responsibility.
- For there to be joint authorship and ownership of strategic planning, deployment of resources and monitoring as well as the development of guidelines and protocols at national, regional and local level by all groups of care givers and women. This can be achieved by including user representatives on groups at all levels and consulting formally. The MSLC is well-placed at district health authority level

to achieve multidisciplinary consultation and ownership of decisions involving all stakeholders (Lewison, 1994).

- There are examples of maternity services user groups composed of women from diverse backgrounds and cultures being consulted informally at local level about changes in maternity services (National Childbirth Trust, 1994). These have tremendous potential for continuing consultation with recent users of the services.

- By keeping the focus on care that is both woman-centred and evidence-based, conflicts are likely to be kept to a minimum.

- Not fearing conflict but regarding it as an opportunity for honest interchange and, possibly, an objective reappraisal, in partnership with women, of the system of care and a positive force for change.

References

Burns, E. (1993). Pooling information. *Nursing Times*, **89** (8): 47–49.

Chapman, V. (1994). Waterbirths: breakthrough or burden? *Br. J. Midwifery*, **2** (1): 17–19.

Department of Health (1993). *Changing Childbirth. The Report of the Expert Maternity Group*. HMSO.

Department of Health (1994). *The Patient's Charter. Maternity Services*. HMSO.

Department of Health (1995). *The Patient's Charter*. HMSO.

Fawdry, R. (1994). Antenatal casenotes 2: general comments. *Br. J. Midwifery*, **2** (8), 371–374.

Galloway, L. S. (1994). Self completion of notes. MIDIRS. *Midwifery Digest*, **4** (2), p. 163.

Garcia, J. and Garforth, S. (1989). Labour and delivery routines in English consultant maternity units. *Midwifery*, **5** (4), 155–162.

Green, J. M., Coupland, V. A. and Kitzinger, J. M. (1990). Expectations, experiences and psychological outcomes of childbirth: a prospective study of 825 women. *Birth*, **17** (1), 15–24.

Health Select Committee (1992). *Winterton Report: Maternity Services. Second Report of the House of Commons Health Committee*. Vol. 1 HMSO, 29–I.

International Confederation of Midwives (1993). *International Code of Ethics for Midwives*. (Available from ICM, 10 Barley Mow Passage, London W4 4PH.)

Kirkham, M. (1989). Midwives and information giving during labour. In *Midwives Research and Childbirth*, Vol. 1 (S. Robinson and A. Thomson, eds). Chapman and Hall.

Lewison, H. (1994). *Maternity Services Liaison Committees. A Forum for Change*. Greater London Association of Community Health Councils.

National Childbirth Trust (1994). *The challenge of change*. (Available from NCT (Maternity Sales) Limited, Burnfield Avenue, Glasgow G46 7TL.)

NHS Management Executive (1994). *Woman centred services*. EL(94)9.

Royal College of Midwives (1994). *The use of water during birth. Position statement*. RCM.

Re S (1992). *All England Law Reports*, **4**, 671–672.

Symon, A. (1994). Midwives and litigation 2: a small-scale survey of attitudes. *Br. J. Midwifery*, **2** (4), 176–181.

UKCC (1993). *Midwives Rules*.

UKCC (1994a). *The Midwife's Code of Practice*.

UKCC (1994b). *Position Statement on Waterbirths*.

Chapter 3

Failure to deliver: Ethical issues relating to epidural analgesia in uncomplicated labour

Rosemary Mander

Introduction: A historical analogy

> The outstanding event in the history of pain relief in childbirth was the first administration of ether for a delivery by Doctor (later Sir) James Young Simpson in Edinburgh in January 1847 (Moir, 1973).

While not underestimating Simpson's achievement in overcoming the opposition of an entrenched medical establishment to the alleviation of a woman's pain in labour, the introduction of this form of pain control was not totally harm-free. This is apparent from contemporaneous accounts of chloroform analgesia reducing uterine activity, which was associated with prolonged labour as well as other, more life-threatening, hazards (Smith, 1979). These adverse side-effects clearly did not manifest themselves in the postprandial research undertaken at Simpson's dinner table. Despite this, chloroform analgesia was generally accepted, to the extent that by thirteen years later it was 'almost universally employed' (Smith, 1979).

The introduction of epidural analgesia into the birthing room just over a century later has certain features in common with the advent of ether and chloroform. These similarities go far beyond the intended effect of pain control, they even go beyond the pharmacological side-effect of weakening uterine contractions. Both of these innovations have contributed to the transfer of control over the birth from the mother to her medical attendant. Both innovations involve a perceived ideal solution by medical practitioners to the problem of pain in labour. Each of these innovations carried with it certain advantages for both mother and obstetrician; each also carried a plethora of side-effects which for the mother would have been hazards, had they not also presented the obstetrician with both reason and opportunity to extend and utilize their rapidly developing interventive skills. Similarly, epidural analgesia comprised a technique which offered for the obstetric anaesthetist an entrée to the birthing room and a route to achieve recognition and professional status (Mander, 1993b).

The use of epidural analgesia in uncomplicated labour, like the less well-documented effects of ether and choloroform, raises a number of issues, many of them carrying serious ethical implications. As I have mentioned already, when such forms of pain control are used, the woman's control over her birth experience is markedly reduced; this has been described in pathophysiological terms (Jouppila et al., 1980; Williams et al., 1985) and is recognized as an example of the 'cascade of intervention' (Varney Burst, 1983). Chloroform analgesia was associated with a reduction in uterine activity and this, together with greater feasibility, increased the incidence of instrumental intervention for the birth (Tew, 1995). In the context of epidural analgesia, the cascade of intervention involves the weakening of uterine contractions as well as certain neurological changes which decrease the tone of the pelvic floor, leading to incomplete rotation of the presenting part, that is, the fetal head in uncomplicated labour. Oxytocic drugs, utilized to overcome the associated delay in labour, increase the risk of fetal hypoxia and the need for instrumental or even surgical intervention for the birth (Yudkin, 1979; Keirse and Chalmers, 1989; Evans, 1992).

Autonomy

The reduction in or loss of bodily control over her labour may also apply at a higher, more intellectual level, in that the mother's control over her personal decision-making, that is her autonomy, may equally be under threat. The challenge to the mother's autonomy derives from the series of events or 'cascade' which may follow the administration of epidural analgesia.

In a child-bearing situation, the various participants may be regarded, or regard themselves, as requiring some degree of autonomy. The balance of autonomy has been observed to be changing for our medical colleagues since the consumerist approach has become a threat to their self-determination (Pellegrino, 1994). Similarly, in association with certain governmental initiatives (House of Commons, 1992; Department of Health, 1993), the midwife may find it necessary to negotiate a *modus vivendi* with the mother to ensure that both retain a mutually acceptable degree of autonomy (Mander, 1993a). The mother's autonomy has recently assumed greater significance due to cultural developments, such as consumerism and the women's movement, and due to organizational changes within the UK health care system, such as the Patient's Charter. The ability of health care systems such as the UK National Health Service to meet the mother's need for autonomy and to provide 'choice in childbirth' has long been questioned (Richards, 1982; Mander, 1993c).

In health care situations, such as child-bearing, the priority that we attach to autonomy leads us to apply it in the form of the ethical principle of respect for autonomy. Such respect manifests itself in our encouragement of autonomous decision-making by clients and patients, an essential feature of which, clearly founded on and arising out of respect for autonomy, is consent to treatment.

Subliminal effects

In considering the elements that create an environment in which 'autonomous authorization' is feasible, Beauchamp and Childress (1989) begin by dismissing competence as a threshold requirement on largely practical grounds. The other two salient components of consent are voluntariness and information. It is necessary for us to consider how these two salient elements may be threatened in the context of epidural analgesia in uncomplicated labour. The concept of coercion is rendered relevant in the present context by the 'subtle threats of ill consequences if ... they do not submit to a recommended course of action' (Beauchamp and Childress, 1989). These subtle threats need not be externally applied. The labour pains that a mother experiences may lead her to anticipate 'ill consequences' in the form of yet more unbearable pain if she declines the analgesic method that may be being dangled tantalizingly in front of her.

Only marginally less subtle is the way in which midwives and other relatively intimate carers may influence the mother's decision-making in labour. This influence may exert its effect in any number of different ways, but possibly by slanting the way in which the available choices are presented. This effective limitation of the mother's decision-making may be regarded as quite a subtle form of coercion. Evidence to support this suggestion is currently merely anecdotal, having been observed by chance during a large and authoritative study of mothers' experience of epidural analgesia (S. Perry, 1993, personal communication). Mothers being cared for by certain individual midwives were found to be consistently either more or less likely to choose epidural analgesia. It may be that Perry's anecdotal observation may be derived from other factors, unrelated to the midwife's personality, attitudes or behaviour. The phenomenon observed by Perry may, alternatively, have been associated with the mother's chance perception of benefits. Further alternative explanations are that certain midwives may have been systematically allocated to care for more 'epidural-prone' mothers or that some midwives may be less well able to cope with the mother's pain or with her way of articulating her pain. It is not possible to assess which of these underlying factors applies without the collection of further data. Perry's observation of the carer's contribution, though, is supported by our knowledge of the limited objectivity in their administration of analgesic agents. These decisions have been clearly shown to be subjective and vulnerable to stereotyping (McDonald, 1994).

Such influence, pressure or coercion by nursing/midwifery staff has, however, been clearly demonstrated in the context of a different intervention in child-bearing. The objectivity of clinical decision-making in relation to Caesarean section (CS) has been called into question (Enkin, 1989). Against this background Radin *et al.* (1993) used a retrospective research design to study the CS rates among 31 labour ward nurses in a north American hospital.

The nurses were categorized according to the CS rates among their healthy, nulliparous 'patients' in spontaneous labour. These researchers found a consistent variation between the nurses in the proportion of 'low-risk' mothers in their care who gave birth by CS. The CS rates of the individual nurses varied between 4·9% and 19% of the mothers for whom each nurse cared. These differences could not be accounted for in the age, parity, socio-economic status, physician in attendance, epidural use, acceleration of labour, stage of labour, baby's weight or gestational age.

The patients of those nurses least associated with CS were also less likely to have a vaginal birth assisted by instruments or a long labour. The lower rates of interventive birth were found not to be associated with any fetal/neonatal ill-effects. The researchers do, however, link these outcomes with the increased likelihood of the nurses with low CS rates obtaining and utilizing psychosocial data about the mothers in their care; this suggests that these nurses took a more woman-oriented approach to care, which may have reinforced the mother's confidence and enabled her to labour physiologically.

Contrary to my earlier suggestion that certain midwives may be systematically allocated to care for certain 'types' of mothers, Radin and her colleagues (Radin *et al.*, 1993) could find no consistent organizational factor that would explain the difference between the nurses' CS rates.

Similarly, more direct association between individual midwives and high or low intervention rates is well-established. A study of midwives' episiotomy rates clearly showed the association between an individual midwife's care and the likelihood of the mother sustaining this form of deliberate perineal damage (Wilkerson, 1984). She reviewed the birth records of 2933 mothers who were cared for at the birth in one unit by any one of 21 midwives during a 12-month-period. This figure constitutes 56·4% of the births in the maternity unit concerned; the remaining births were medically supervised. Each midwife was identified by a letter of the alphabet, in order of their frequency of performing an episiotomy.

The chances of the mother sustaining an episiotomy varied hugely. A mother being cared for by 'Midwife A' was over ten times more likely to encounter this form of perineal damage than her sister who was being cared for by 'Midwife U'. Of the primigravidae cared for by 'Midwife A', 92·8% sustained an episiotomy, whereas only 3% of multigravidae cared for by 'Midwife U' sustained one.

While the huge variation in midwives' practice is apparent from Wilkerson's data, it is necessary to question why midwives like 'Midwife A' practised in such a 'scissor-happy', though far from unique, manner (Inch, 1982). Protecting the integrity of the pelvic floor and the fetal brain have been cited as the rationale for episiotomy, but changing attitudes may have been more significant. Attitudes are likely to have been influenced by midwives' own statutory bodies, the Central Midwives Boards, who in 1967 incorporated perineal infiltration and episiotomy into midwifery training. A further influence was the surgical orientation of midwives' medical colleagues (Wilkerson, 1984), which increased the pressure on midwives to intervene in this way. This pressure carried with it serious implications for mothers' autonomy and midwives' decision-making as evidenced by the emergence of the 'routine prophylactic episiotomy' (Formato, 1985).

Episiotomy is clearly a particularly direct example of midwives' influence over interventions. It is necessary to consider the possibility of more subtle pressure such as those used in episiotomy. The more subtle effects have been shown in both the research-based observations relating to CS and the more anecdotal evidence concerning epidural analgesia, mentioned above.

Midwives' insider knowledge

As well as the voluntariness of the mother's decision being influenced more or less subliminally by the midwife's attitudes and information-giving, the decision may also be influenced by the midwife's specialist knowledge. The mother's decision to accept or not to accept an offer of epidural analgesia may be affected by the midwife's knowledge of the person who will be 'siting', that is inserting into the epidural space, the epidural cannula and local anaesthetic. The midwife may be aware of the level of the technical skills of the obstetric anaesthetist on call. Even obstetric anaesthetists admit the existence of and dangers associated with the practice of unskilled anaesthetists (Morgan, 1987), so it is hardly surprising that midwives may come to question the standard of the technical expertise of some of their anaesthetist colleagues. Clearly, a midwife's ability to encourage a mother in her care to accept epidural analgesia is likely to be influenced by the midwife's assessment, based on previous observational experience, of the expertise of the practitioner who is on call at the relevant time. In the same way that the midwife may seek to protect the mother in her care from an unskilled anaesthetist, she may similarly seek to protect the mother from an unsatisfactory interpersonal encounter. While the siting of an epidural cannula may not be an intensely painful procedure, it is not always easy for a mother in labour to remain still and in a suitable position. As one mother told Oakley

(1993): 'I found it very hard to keep still on my side in labour with needles being put in my back. Especially when a pain came.'

A certain amount of coaxing and encouragement by the anaesthetist may be necessary. While the communication skills of the obstetric anaesthetist may make this arduous procedure easier and less tiresome, some anaesthetists may lack the high level of interpersonal skills necessary to achieve this. The midwife may judge that the likelihood of a disturbing interpersonal encounter for the mother may not be justified in view of the level of pain that she perceives the mother to be facing and, thus, she may discourage her implicitly or openly from choosing epidural analgesia.

Thus, the midwife's knowledge of the personnel likely to be involved may influence the 'voluntariness' of the mother's epidural decision.

Pressure of bias

Draper (1991) links coercion with the way in which information is presented to the client or patient. Draper's examples include, first, the order in which the various options are recounted to the mother, although she does not indicate whether those higher on the list are more likely to be favoured or vice versa. Second, Draper explains how pressure may be applied by unduly emphasizing either the benefits of a certain, favoured, course of action or the hazards or damaging side-effects of the less favourable course of action. Information given to the mother relating to epidural analgesia may employ both of these strategies; an example of the latter use of emphasis is found in an informational booklet distributed to all mothers in one National Health Trust: 'Epidurals do not cause sleepiness in the baby in the same way as an injection of diamorphine or pethidine' (Stewart and West, undated).

By way of support for Draper's comments, the use of the 'hard sell' to persuade the mother to accept epidural analgesia has been observed and reported by campaigning organizations, some of which attempt to preserve the mother's control over her birth experience by ensuring the voluntariness of her decision-making (Robinson, 1993).

Expectation of failure

As in many situations in life and in some relating to child-bearing, women learn at an early stage of the risk of failure. The mother's voluntary decision-making may be limited by pressure deriving from the expectation of failure. If this expectation is held, however unconsciously, by those near her, it may undermine the confidence of the mother. As Tew (1995) observes, confidence is fundamentally important to successful, physiological child-bearing. She suggests that obstetricians have sought to establish their professional status by winning public confidence through 'destroying the confidence of mothers in their own reproductive efficiency'. Tew observes that the confidence of other carers, such as midwives, was also destroyed. This undermining of women's self-confidence began with the introduction of antenatal care in the early years of the 20th century (Tew, 1995). A similar strategy was employed to persuade mothers and midwives of the 'total safety' of hospital birth (Beech, 1992).

Particularly vulnerable is the mother's confidence in her own ability to labour successfully and physiologically. The expectation of failure to cope with the physiological processes of labour is shared by staff as well as mothers and has resulted in the 'hard sell' mentioned above (Robinson, 1993).

Another example of the expectation of failure would be the traditional 'education' about breast feeding, which features details of the associated problems, such as breast engorgement, cracked nipples, inadequate milk supply and mastitis (Blumfield, 1992). Such 'education' tends to be provided alongside details of formula feeding (Watson and Mander, 1995). In this way, the mother's confidence in her ability to breast feed is undermined, while a less healthy message is transmitted through supposedly health promotional material.

The expectation of failure may be held by a variety of formal and informal carers with whom the mother is in contact prior to and during her labour. These carers or agents may be, for convenience, divided into four groups: the formal carers, the informal carers, policy makers and other mothers.

The formal carers: Midwives and medical staff

The differing expectations became apparent in a research project undertaken by Walker (1972, 1976), which distiguished the approaches of midwives and their medical colleagues. The midwives were clearly able to assume a waiting role during labour, in the expectation that, given time, nature would effectively take its course and result in a healthy outcome. The medical staff, on the other hand, regarded every labour as potentially pathological until it was safely completed, thus requiring their personal supervision, availability and enthusiasm for intervention at all times. The medical expectation of failure in child-bearing has been summarized by Percival (1970) in his oft-quoted aphorism: 'Labour is only normal in retrospect.'

It may be, because obstetricians during their training are unlikely to observe more than a small number of normal labours and in the course of their practice none at all, that they have difficulty anticipating a physiological outcome to labour. In the same way, obstetric anaesthetists tend not to be involved with a mother who is coping well with her pain in labour, and thus may have difficulty envisaging the prospect of an unmedicated labour. In addition to their other reasons for advocating the increasing use of epidural analgesia in uncomplicated labour (Mander, 1993b), limited experience of women coping may engender in obstetric anaesthetists the expectation of failure to cope.

Informal and cultural influences

While clearly apparent in some situations, the expectation of failure to cope with pain in labour may not operate in certain other cultures. Such a culture, which has been the focus of considerable interest and some research attention, is the Netherlands. It is generally assumed that the Dutch mother's ability to cope with labour pain unassisted by medication is learned behaviour which may be culturally determined; as Tasharrofi (1993) observes, the result is that analgesia is 'neither expected nor required'. The important cultural component in the acceptance or otherwise of labour pain has been attributed to some cultures' adherence to the medical model of health (van Teijlingen, 1994).

To illustrate this differing orientation, Senden and colleagues (1988) undertook a study comparing the expectations and experiences of labour pain in mothers in Iowa (USA) and Nijmegen (Netherlands). In a sample of 256 mothers, a large majority of Dutch mothers (79·2%) did not use medication to control labour pain, whereas this applied to only 37·6% of American mothers. The proportions in each group showing satisfaction with their method of pain control and the fulfilment of their expectations of pain showed no significant differences. These authors consider that their findings reflect attitudes which are derived from the confidence of Dutch women, learned through personal, family and social experience, in their own ability to cope with labour pain and to labour successfully.

Policy factors

A further factor, not unrelated to the previous two, which may be involved in the way in which the mother's expectation of failure may limit the voluntariness of her decision-making is the organizational aspects of her child-bearing experience as determined by local and national health policy. By this I mean the location of childbirth for the vast majority of mothers in the UK – the hospital.

Inevitably, and probably correctly, hospitalization carries with it an aura of illness, which is transposed to the physiological process of child-bearing. Thus, birth is transformed into a potentially pathological process and in need of safety precautions, possibly in the form of medical interventions, to prevent dire consequences. Macfarlane (1992) maintains that the safety argument is founded on the observation that mortality rates are currently lower than they were when home birth was more easily available and happened more generally. As a result, she argues, hospital birth is assumed to be the *cause* of lower mortality rates. In this way the notion of safety is used to justify the currently high hospital birth rates and to intimidate women into giving birth in hospital (Beech, 1991). Hence, organizational factors raise the expectation of failure in the mother and further limit the voluntariness of her decision-making.

Other mothers' 'old wives' tales'

Personal observation leads me to believe that mothers themselves may encourage in each other the expectation of failure. This is through phenomena which have been referred to as 'old wives' tales' and 'new wives' tales' (Perkins, 1980). These are the traditional, as well as more modern, horror stories which mothers have since time immemorial shared with mothers-to-be. My own observation indicates that 'old wives' tales' not infrequently focus on labour pain. This focus emphasizes the severity, the duration and the irremediable nature of this pain. These stories clearly serve to help the mother relating the tale to adjust to her experience of childbirth and may help her to restore her self-esteem after what she may perceive to have been a disappointing and degrading experience. The benefits, however, for the mother-to-be are less obvious and may serve to arouse in her the expectation of failure to cope.

Taking a broader view, we see that the expectation of failure features prominently in the folklore of childbirth. While the prospect of maternal death has thankfully receded, the spectres of other failures have assumed greater significance. These spectres have been used to advantage by certain groups to achieve ends which are not solely for the benefit of the mother and her baby. The specialty of obstetric anaesthesia, initially introduced to solve the problem of an intransigent maternal death rate, has developed into a profession by fostering in mothers the expectation of their inability to cope with the pain of uncomplicated labour and by offering an intervention to prevent that pain (Mander, 1993b, 1994). Through the modification of mothers' expectations and the development and maintenance of a professional group, on both an individual and a cultural basis, the widespread use of epidural analgesia has served to limit the voluntary decision-making or autonomy of child-bearing women.

Information

The demarcation between obtaining consent and giving adequate information is not always easily distinguishable; this is because consent, unless preceded by giving the patient or client relevant information, is worthless. Lindley (1991) spells out the possible repercussions for the practitioner in terms of first, being guilty of battery and second, rendering the practitioner open to claims for damages. He maintains that such claims would be likely to be upheld regardless of whether the patient was injured, whether the practitioner was negligent or whether consent would have been forthcoming had it been sought.

The standard of information-giving may be measured according to the professional practice standard, the reasonable person standard or the subjective standard (Beauchamp and Childress, 1989; Henderson, 1994).

Quality of the information relating to epidural analgesia

The quantity of the information that is given to the patient or client varies according to which of the above standards is operating. The quality of that information may also vary according to an even broader range of determinants. This may be seen to apply in the context of epidural analgesia in uncomplicated labour. The quality of the information may be affected by exogenous factors, such as the existence or non-existence of relevant research or may be biased by endogenous factors such as personal and professional attitudes.

The research basis

As in so many aspects of maternity care the research evidence on which our practice is based is far from adequate and does not enable the mother to give fully informed consent to her care (Chalmers, 1993). The lack of authoritative research evidence places the midwife and, more importantly, the mother in a quandary about the most appropriate care for mother and baby. Richards (1982) observes that, like many interventions in child-bearing, epidural analgesia was introduced for the benefit of a small number of women to avoid serious, that is life-threatening, problems. On the basis of positive experiences for these few women, and without the benefit of randomized controlled trials of its efficacy, this form of pain control was made available to large numbers of mothers experiencing uncomplicated childbirth (Chalmers, 1993). This medical logic was summarized succinctly by Baird *et al.* (1953): 'If it is accepted that [this intervention] is safer for certain types of patient where the risks are high, it must also be safer where the risks are less.' Like research into the benefits and hazards of other frequently used interventions in child-bearing, such as ultrasound, after approximately 30 years of widespread use it is becoming too late to put the genie back into the bottle. The research that was neglected when these techniques were in their infancy may no longer be feasible.

The research evidence that is available is limited in its scope, being largely confined to the technical aspects of epidural analgesia, and not well utilized in practice. This is apparent in a booklet for mothers which, while advocating the epidural, fails to mention practically the only research evidence on this topic about which there is 'confidence' (Howell and Chalmers, 1992). Mention of the increased use of instruments to assist the birth is omitted, with barely passing, but reassuring reference, to second-stage delay: 'During the second stage of labour the urge to "bear down" may be reduced, but your midwife is trained to help you bear down when it is appropriate' (Stewart and West, undated).

The general lack of relevant research-based information is apparent in a number of crucial areas relating to epidural analgesia in uncomplicated labour.

Long-term effects

Partly because the mother's stay in the maternity unit is becoming shorter and partly because her care lacks continuity, the long-term effects of epidural analgesia in labour have passed largely unnoticed. Sheila Kitzinger's (1987) methodologically odd study was the first to draw our attention to the neurological and orthopaedic sequelae of epidural analgesia in uncomplicated labour (Mander, 1994). Although large ($n = 908$), Kitzinger's sample comprised NCT volunteers in the UK and Australia. The sample was self-selected, uncontrolled and, presumably, highly motivated. There were approximately equal numbers from each country. Drawing on the experiences of this sample in a qualitative research design, Kitzinger reports an epidural failure rate of 15%, as well as more serious problems such as sudden hypotensive episodes and dural tap. She mentions that 18% of the sample perceived themselves to be suffering from long-term side-effects including neurological and orthopaedic symptoms. The emotional sequelae, such as regrets and feelings of failure, were found to be delayed for weeks, months or even until the birth of the next baby.

While Kitzinger's research project may obviously be criticized for the selection of the sample, the researcher makes no unjustified claims about the generalizability of her conclusions. She does not use the term, but her work indicates the existence of the 'cascade of intervention' in the experiences of her informants.

The reception accorded to the far more authoritative study by MacArthur and her colleagues (1992) was barely more accepting of the incapacitating and enduring effects of this form of pain control. Despite the findings of MacArthur *et al.* being initially disregarded for sampling reasons and their veracity being denied, they have been accepted, albeit reluctantly (Robinson, 1993).

The original aim of MacArthur and her colleagues was to study the long-term health implications of pregnancy and child-bearing (1992). This retrospective study was large and the sampling and methodological detail is comprehensive. The data illuminate the wide-ranging, pervasive and enduring health problems following childbirth. The data on the long-term health sequelae associated with the use of epidural analgesia in labour are consistent with Kitzinger's findings (1987).

MacArthur and her colleagues found that 19·3% of mothers who gave birth vaginally while using epidural analgesia developed long-term backache; whereas only 10·4% of those mothers who gave birth vaginally without epidural analgesia did so. For some mothers who had used epidural analgesia, the backache was accompanied by headache, migraine, shoulder/neckaches, pain/weakness of limbs or tingling of the extremities.

The hypothesis advanced by MacArthur is that these neurological and orthopaedic sequelae are associated with sublinical trauma to the 'spinal axis' during labour. She maintains that the minor discomforts which ordinarily cause a person to adjust their posture are neither perceptible nor correctable under the effect of epidural analgesia. These trauma later manifest themselves as symptoms due to the superimposed stress of caring for a young baby.

This debate was joined by MacLeod et al. (1995) who contributed data collected prior to the media attention attracted by MacArthur's work. These obstetric anaesthetists surveyed 2065 mothers one year after the birth and achieved a 67·1% response rate. Of the mothers who had used epidural analgesia, 26·2% were found to have developed new long-term backache since the birth. Of those mothers not exposed to epidural analgesia, only 1·7% developed backache.

The use to which these research findings have been put may not accord with the intentions of the researchers, in that, as Robinson observes, informing a mother who is not coping with her labour pain that, 'An epidural could cause you long term backache—do you still want it?' may not be the most appropriate use of this information (Robinson, 1993).

Mother-oriented concerns

The limited research attention focused on the concerns of mothers relating to pain control methods compares dismally with the generous research attention to issues relating to the technique of administering epidural analgesia (Mander, 1994). It is necessary to question whether this focus reflects the medical view of research in more general terms. The 'scientific' approach espoused by our medical colleagues values the measurement of phenomena, such as physiological observations. Such measurements carry the reassuring certainty that they are incontrovertible and, thus, valued. The reverse may equally apply, to the extent that phenomena that are not measurable may be denied, disregarded or dismissed as of no value. For these reasons mothers' responses to pain control have been given only superficial research attention, and have sought largely to persuade the active birth movement of the errors of its ways (Mander, 1994).

Researchers who have undertaken authoritative studies into the mother's feelings and expectations during child-bearing indicate that perceptions of being in control are crucial to the mother's satisfaction with her experience (Green *et al.*, 1990). The effects of the method of pain control on the mother's perception of control also require research attention; this would enable carers to give to the mother who wishes to retain control during childbirth the information that would allow her to do so (Mander, 1992). Oakley (1993), in her follow up to a major research project, admittedly identifies how much the effectiveness of epidural analgesia is appreciated by mothers. She endorses Green's findings, though, by observing that mothers are far less satisfied with their feelings of diminished control, together with other side-effects and long-term health problems.

In her conclusion Oakley (1993) reports the integrated view that mothers adopt of their birth experience, including the pain. She regrets that researchers are less able to reflect this holistic view of birth, tending to make measurements and ask simplistic questions about satisfaction. The researcher's distinction between physical and emotional phenomena does not appear to match the mother's experience. Oakley argues that the research orientation needs to be adapted in order to combine emotional as well as physical aspects of pain. In this way it may become possible to provide the mother with the information that she needs before consenting to an intervention such as epidural analgesia.

Failure rates

An example of information with physical and emotional implications which needs to be made available to mothers, prior to valid decisions being made about pain control in labour, is the local success rate. This aspect of epidural analgesia is not considered serious enough to warrant publication, even less, research attention (Crawford, 1986). Writing about non-pharmacological methods of pain control, Simkin (1989) briefly indicates the success rates of lumbar epidural analgesia as being between 67 and 90%. Additionally, one of the few studies even to mention the possibility of epidural failure is the much-criticized work by Kitzinger (1987), which reports an epidural failure rate of 15%.

The reason for my plea for more research-based information on this topic lies in the serious implications of a failed epidural for the mother and for her carers. In this situation the mother is likely to have prepared herself for a little discomfort, but certainly not for the full-blown pain of labour. Despite the best efforts of our anaesthetist colleagues the problem may not be resolved. Not surprisingly I have found the mother in this situation to be disappointed and angry, as well as suffering pain for which she has not prepared herself either physically or emotionally. As a midwife I have to draw on my full repertoire of caring and interpersonal skills to support the mother through this doubly negative experience.

The difficulty that anaesthetists encounter in facing the possibility of a failed epidural was impressed on me on one such occasion. The most senior anaesthetist had been summoned to resolve the apparently intractable problem of an unsupported mother's failed epidural. In response to this dismal scenario, she asked the miserable, frightened and angry young mother: 'Why are you making all this fuss? I had four without an epidural and I never made all this noise.'

Professional factors

As well as factors relating to the existence of appropriate information about epidural analgesia, we need to consider how and whether such information as exists is transmitted to the mother for her use. Inevitably, the information in this context is largely unidirectional, that is, from the practitioner to the mother.

Paternalism, which has been mentioned already, may operate alone or, in certain situations, may become entangled with professional relationships to affect information-giving. These relationships may be inter-professional, inter-occupational or client-professional. Regardless of the personnel involved, there are serious implications for the transmission of information and, eventually, decision-making.

Inter-occupational relationships have been shown by Kirkham (1989) to influence adversely information-giving by personnel and occupational groups perceived as being of different status. Kirkham's finding was that, in the presence of colleagues perceived to be of higher status, carers were less likely to inform the labouring mother of choices and developments. Because the higher-status staff do not consider such information-giving as part of their remit, the mother found herself even less well informed since the arrival of the 'expert'.

The implications of 'medical dominance' for the operation of consent in a general surgical setting were researched by Meredith (1993). Because of their poor impressions of the intellectual abilities of their patients 'the surgeons . . . were not enthusiastic at the prospect of devoting more time to discussing surgical alternatives, risks and complications, and outlook indicators for their patient's benefit.' It may be that, in child-bearing, medical dominance may be less oppressive due to the absence of illness from the equation. The contribution of illness, however, is probably small, if it exists, but of far greater significance is the part played by power relationships (Freidson, 1970). He suggests that even though terms such as 'professional' have become devalued by wider educational opportunities, their underlying feature remains unchanged; this feature is power. In this context power relates to the ability to control one's work through education and legislation as well as on a more mundane basis, by controlling the 'market' within which one operates. Despite the recent reforms in the UK health care system, it is clear that power, as defined by Freidson, has been retained by medics to a far greater extent than by other health care providers or by health care consumers. Freidson questions whether in future this power may be worth less, due to the increasing specialization of industries, which may include health care. He considers, optimistically, that the increasing fragmentation of the professions will give rise to a need for cooperation between the differing occupational groups and, inevitably, the consumer. Thus, the mother's input into decision-making is likely to increase if this scenario materializes.

Conclusion

I have questioned the ethical basis upon which epidural services are provided for the mother experiencing uncomplicated labour. Certain organizational and occupational factors have been shown to reduce the likelihood of the mother being able to give valid consent. This likelihood is further reduced by the lack of appropriate research-based information and the limited willingness of those involved to impart such relevant information as does exist.

Throughout this chapter the possibility of failure has featured prominently. The acceptance of epidural services has been fostered by the expectation that mothers will fail to cope with the pain of uncomplicated labour.

The development of epidural services has not been supported by research into those areas of pain control which are likely to to be of concern to mothers, such as success rates, long-term side-effects and non-life-threatening side-effects. Thus, the informational needs of the mother are not satisfied sufficiently to permit her to decide on and give valid consent to the most appropriate form of pain control. Significant among the information on epidural analgesia that has not been provided are the failure rates of this intervention.

While decisions about the introduction of innovative methods of pain control for use in labour may, in the past, have been made in fashionable Edinburgh dining rooms, such 'research' is no longer adequate. Before the mother is able to give valid consent, that is fully informed consent, to interventions such as epidural analgesia, certain requirements need to be satisfied. The first is that the mother is aware of her physiological, psychological and emotional states and can make decisions as to whether she is able to cope with the pain of uncomplicated labour. The second is that she is aware of the implications of such interventions, for herself in the short and long term, for her labour, as well as for her baby. These implications inevitably include the possibility of the intervention failing to meet her expectations.

References

Baird, D., Thomson, A. and Duncan, E. (1953). The causes and prevention of stillbirths and first week deaths; Part II: Evidence from Aberdeen clinical records. *J. Obstet. Gynaecol.*, **60**, 17–30.

Beauchamp, T. L. and Childress, J. F. (1989). *Principles of Biomedical Ethics*, 3rd edn. Oxford University Press.

Beech, B. L. (1991). Home birth: What kind of choice? *AIMS Q. J.*, 3 (2), 6–7.

Beech, B. L. (1992). Women's Views of Childbirth, Chapter 11. In *Obstetrics in the 1990s: Current Controversies* (Chard, T. and Richard, M. P. M.) MacKeith Press.

Blumfield, W. (1992). *Life After Birth: Every Woman's Guide to the First Year of Motherhood*. Element Books, Shaftesbury.

Chalmers, I. (1993). Effective care in midwifery: Research, the professions and the public. *Midwives Chronicle*, 106 (1260), 3–12.

Crawford, J. S. (1986). Some maternal complications of epidural analgesia for labour. *Obstet. Anaesthes. Dig.*, 6 (2), 221–222.

Department of Health (1993). *Changing Childbirth: Report of the Expert Maternity Group*. HMSO.

Doughty, A. (1987). Landmarks in the development of regional analgesia in obstetrics. In *Foundations of Obstetric Anaesthesia* (B. M. Morgan, ed.) Farrand Press.

Draper, H. (1991). Sterilization abuse: Women and consent to treatment. In *Protecting the Vulnerable: Autonomy and Consent in Health Care* (M. Brazier and M. Lobjoit, eds), pp. 77–100, Routledge.

Enkin, M. (1989). Commentary: Why do the Caesarean section rates differ? *Birth*, 16, 207–208.

Evans, S. (1992). The value of cardiotocograph monitoring in midwifery. *Midwives Chronicle*, 105 (1248), 4–11.

Formato, L.-S. (1985). Routine prophylactic episiotomy. *J. Nurse-Midwifery*, 30 (3), pp. 144–148.

Freidson, E. (1970). *Profession of Medicine*. Mead & Co.

Green, J. M., Coupland, V. A. and Kitzinger, J. V. (1990). Expectations, experiences and psychological outcomes of childbirth: A prospective study of 825 women. *Birth*, 17 (1), 15–24.

Henderson, M. (1994). Risk and the doctor–patient relationship. In *Principles of Health Care Ethics* (R. Gillon and A. Lloyd, eds), pp. 435–444. John Wiley & Sons.

House of Commons (1992). *Health Committee Second Report, Maternity Services*. HMSO.

Howell, C. J. and Chalmers, I. (1992). A review of prospectively controlled comparisons of epidural with non-epidural forms of pain relief during labour. *Int. J. Obstet. Anaesthes.*, 1, 93–110.

Inch, S. (1982). *Birthrights*. Hutchinson.

Jouppila, R., Jouppila, P., Moilanen, K. and Pakarinen, A. (1980). The effect of segmental epidural analgesia on maternal prolactin during labour. *Br. J. Obstet. Gynaecol.*, 31 (1), 1–10.

Keirse, M. J. N. C. and Chalmers, I. (1989). Methods for inducing labour, Ch. 62. In *Effective Care in Pregnancy and Childbirth*, Vol. 2: *Childbirth* (I. Chalmers, M. Enkin and M. J. N. C. Keirse, eds), pp. 1057–79. Oxford University Press.

Kirkham, M. (1989). Midwives and information-giving during labour. In *Midwives, Research and Childbirth* (S. Robinson and A. M. Thomson, eds). Chapman & Hall.

Kitzinger, S. (1987). *Some Women's Experiences of Epidurals—a Descriptive Study*. National Childbirth Trust.

Lindley, R. (1991). Informed consent and the ghost of Bolam. In *Protecting the Vulnerable: Autonomy and Consent in Health Care* (M. Brazier and M. Lobjoit, eds), pp. 134–149, Routledge.

MacArthur, C. (1991). *Health After Childbirth*, HMSO.

MacArthur, C., Lewis, M. and Knox, E. G. (1992). Investigation of long-term problems after obstetric epidural anaesthesia. *Br. Med. J.*, 304, 1279–1282.

Macfarlane, A. (1992). Interpreting statistics. *Nursing Times*, 88 (35), 62.

MacLeod, J., MacIntyre, C., McClure, J. H. and Whitfield, A. (1995). Backache and epidural analgesia. *Int. J. Obstet. Anaesthes.*, 4, 21–25.

Mander, R. (1992). The control of pain in labour. *J. Clin. Nurs.*, 1, 219–223.

Mander, R. (1993a). Autonomy in midwifery and maternity care. *Midwives Chronicle*, 106 (1269), 369–374.

Mander, R. (1993b). Epidural analgesia 1: Recent history. *Br. J. Midwifery*, 1 (6), 259–264.

Mander, R. (1993c). 'Who chooses the choices?' *Modern Midwife*, 3 (1), 23–25.

Mander, R. (1994). Epidural analgesia: 2. Research basis. *Br. J. Midwifery*, 2 (1), 12–16.

McDonald, D. D. (1994). Gender and ethnic stereotyping and narcotic analgesic administration. *Res. Nurs. Health*, 17 (1), 45–49.

Meredith, P. (1993). Patient participation in decision-making and consent to treatment: The case of general surgery. *Sociol. Health Illness*, 15 (3), 315–336.

Moir, D. D. (1973). Pain Relief in Labour: A Handbook for Midwives, 2nd edition, Churchill Livingstone.

Morgan, B. M. (1987). Mortality and anaesthesia. In *Foundations of Obstetric Anaesthesia* (B. M. Morgan, ed.), Farrand Press.

Nicholson, R. (1991). The ethics of research with children. In *Protecting the Vulnerable: Autonomy and Consent in Health Care* (M. Brazier and H. Lobjoit, eds), pp. 10–21. Routledge.

Oakley, A. (1993). The follow-up survey. In *Pain and Its Relief in Childbirth* (G. Chamberlain, A. Wraight and P. Steer), pp. 101–14, Churchill Livingstone.

Pellegrino, E. D. (1994). The four principles and the doctor–patient relationship: the need for a better linkage, Ch. 31. In *Principles of Health Care Ethics* (R. Gillon and A. Lloyd, eds), p. 353, John Wiley & Sons.

Percival, R. C. (1970). Management of normal labour. *The Practitioner*, March Vol. 204, 1221–1224.

Perkins, E. R. (1980). *Education for Childbirth and Parenthood*, Croom Helm.

Radin, T. G., Harmon, J. S. and Hanson, D. A. (1993). Nurses' care during labor: its effect on the Cesarean birth rate of healthy, nulliparous women. *Birth*, 20 (1), 14–21.

Richards, M. P. M. (1982). The trouble with 'choice' in childbirth. *Birth*, 9 (4), 253–260.

Robinson, J. (1993). Long term consequence of epidurals and other childbirth care. *AIMS Q. J.*, 5 (1), 27–28.

Senden, I. P. M., van der Wettering, M. D., Eskes, A. B., *et al.* (1988). Labour pain: A comparison of parturients in a Dutch and an American teaching hospital. *Obstet. Gynecol.*, 71 (4), 451–453.

Simkin, P. (1989). Non-pharmacological methods of pain control. In *Effective Care in Pregnancy and Childbirth*, Vol. 2 (I. Chalmers, M. Enkin and M. J. N. C. Keirse, eds), p. 20, Oxford University Press.

Smith, F. B. (1979). *The People's Health 1830–1910*. Holmes & Meier.

Stewart, M. and West, C. (Undated). *The Birth of Your Baby at the Simpson*,

Tasharrofi, A. (1993). Midwifery care in the Netherlands. *Midwives Chronicle*, 106 (1267), 286–288.

Tew, M. (1995). *Safer Childbirth?: A Critical History of Maternity Care*. Chapman & Hall.

van Teijlingen, E. (1994). A social or medical model of childbirth? Comparing the arguments in Grampian (Scotland) and the Netherlands. Unpublished PhD Thesis, University of Aberdeen.

Varney Burst, H. (1983). The influence of consumers in the birthing movement. *Top. Clin. Nurs.*, 5, 42–54.

Walker, J. (1972). The changing role of the midwife. *Int. J. Nurs. Studies*, 9, 85–94.

Walker, J. (1976). Midwife or obstetric nurse? Some perceptions of midwives and obstetricians of the role of the midwife. *J. Adv. Nurs.*, 1, 129–138.

Watson, N. and Mander, R. (1995). Advertising Infant Formula in the Maternity Area. *MIDIRS Midwifery Digest*, 5 (3), 338–41.

Wilkerson, V. A. (1984). The use of episiotomy in normal delivery. *Midwives Chronicle*, 97 (1155), 106–110.

Williams, S., Hepburn, M. and McIlwaine, G. (1985). Consumer view of epidural anaesthesia. *Midwifery*, 1 (1), 32–36.

Yudkin, P., Frumar, A. M., Anderson, A. B. M. and Turnbull, A. C. (1979). A retrospective study of induction of labour. *Br. J. Obstet. Gynaecol.*, 86 (4), 257–265.

Chapter 4

Ethical issues concerning ultrasound in pregnancy

Jean Proud

Introduction

Ultrasound scanning has become an integral part of antenatal care. Most women expect it and most obstetricians and midwives rely on it to form the basis on which to monitor a pregnancy. The technology has developed at a rapid rate and scanning is increasingly used in the care of all pregnant women. These factors have overtaken any thoughts that might be given to the ethical implications of prenatal screening and this chapter will explore some of these ethical issues. The debate will focus on the validity of routine scanning, considering the amount of information that should be given to women so that they can make an informed choice about scanning, paternalistic practice, whether to tell the truth about scanning results and finally the practical implications of the medical ethic of beneficence will be examined.

Background and development

When Ian Donald first introduced ultrasound into obstetrics in the 1950s, by submerging his subjects in a bath of water, it was used selectively to assess the gestational age of the fetus and to locate the placenta. However, very soon after its introduction as a diagnostic aid for women experiencing problems, for example antepartum haemorrhage, the clinicians began to realize its potential as a screening tool for all pregnant women. In most cases this was introduced according to the utilitarian principle that it would benefit the majority. 'Risk factors' could be identified, for example, the low-lying placenta and for all women an accurate expected date of delivery could be predicted (Warsof *et al.*, 1983).

During the 1970s the grey scale was developed and the images were no longer seen in outline only. This meant various tissues could be differentiated and characterized. As the images improved operators increased their knowledge of fetal anatomy and, consequently, markers of fetal anomalies and disease. The enthusiasm with which this new knowledge was greeted overshadowed warning voices objecting to its ever-increasing use in pregnancy. Among these have been midwives, in particular members of AIMS (Robinson and Beech, 1993). Chervenak and McCullough (1991), addressing the morality of this practice, wrote: 'Ethics is an emerging subdiscipline of obstetric ultrasound because there are clinical dimensions of obstetric ultrasound that only ethics can identify and address.' Walkinshaw in a paper to a symposium in 1992 said that, in his opinion, the ethical issues surrounding ultrasound in pregnancy had never been properly addressed.

The majority of problems with regard to the morality of scanning arise out of its use as a screening procedure. However, one central problem stems from the fact that it is used both as a screening procedure and as a diagnostic tool and sometimes it is difficult or impossible to separate the two. A routine scan offered as a screening procedure can develop into a diagnostic tool as anomalies are discovered, identified and a diagnosis made. At other times, a scan can be used primarily as a diagnostic tool to investigate signs or symptoms of disease in the mother, for example an abdominal pain, but it is possible that, even when it is used for such diagnostic purposes, fetal anomalies can be revealed.

The debate concerning the routine use of ultrasound

The ethical justification for screening programmes, in general, is the utilitarian principle of the end justifying the means. Good actions should produce the greatest happiness for the greatest number and the best possible consequences. Routine scanning is undertaken to predict an accurate date of delivery and to detect the abnormal or the diseased fetus so that action can be taken to improve the outcome, either to eradicate it or offer some form of treatment to correct or cure it. Thus, screening is justified on the grounds that it is for the benefit of the majority of the population screened.

Proponents of deontology would hold that actions are right or wrong apart from any good consequences they produce or bad consequences they prevent; each individual should be treated as an end in themselves, not as a means to an end (as possibly sanctioned by utilitarianism). This incorporates the ethic of caring for the individual, and because it considers the individual it emphasizes the importance of autonomy. Patient autonomy in the area of screening means letting women have a choice, choice over the type of care they want and choice concerning any prenatal tests they might be encouraged to undertake.

Some of the arguments in favour of routine scanning are directed at improving perinatal mortality and morbidity figures. This could be achieved in several ways.

- A pregnancy could be terminated if a fetus is discovered to be suffering from an anomaly and this would result in fewer babies being born with congenital abnormalities and/or genetic disease (Brock et al., 1978; Luck, 1992). (This assumes, of course, that fewer babies with abnormalities is a good thing; see Chapter 8.)
- Mothers expecting babies with less serious problems can receive appropriate antenatal care and, if necessary, be moved to centres of excellence specializing in appropriate neonatal care when their babies are born (Luck, 1992).
- Confirming the gestational age of the fetus by ultrasound improves fetal outcome because it reduces the risks of postmaturity, which, in turn, reduces the risks of prematurity because timing the induction of labour is more accurate (Bennett et al., 1982; Bakketeig et al., 1984; Eik-Nes, 1984; Giersson, 1991).
- Assessing the gestational age of the fetus in the first or second trimester of pregnancy also allows screening for growth problems of the fetus to be monitored more accurately. This ensures that the fetus at risk of growth problems is discovered at an early stage; this can be particularly important in the multiple pregnancy (Grennert et al., 1978; Persson et al., 1979).

Other research casts doubt on the advantages of routine scanning. A randomized controlled trial (Neilson et al., 1984), a large multicentred trial involving 15 151 pregnant women in the United States (Ewigman *et al.*, 1993) and a meta-analysis performed by Bucher and Schmidt (1993), have suggested that there were no significant advantages to the practice of routine scanning in pregnancy in terms of an increased number of live births, an improvement in perinatal outcome for multiple gestations or infants who were small for gestational age. Further, there was no reduction in perinatal morbidity.

Arguments against routine ultrasound in pregnancy state that its use has never been properly evaluated, an issue that was raised by Hall (1991) in her response to the Health of the Nation document. There are also repeated media and journal reports calling for more research into the safety aspects of scanning, suggesting that routine ultrasound examination of pregnant women should cease until such studies have ruled out any possible hazards associated with its use. Salvesen *et al.* (1992) have suggested a possible association of ultrasound scans of the fetus *in utero* with subsequent non-righthandedness of the child, while Newham *et al.* (1993) suggest frequent scanning in pregnancy is associated with subsequent low birth weight. AIMS (1993) published a special issue of their quarterly journal to emphasize a growing concern about the routine use of a technology that has had no formal assessment of the risks, benefits of its use or its levels of safety.

Health care professionals often 'sell' routine scanning to women by telling them it is performed to make sure the 'baby is all right'. The presumption is thus conveyed that if it is not something can be done about it. This approach was criticized by Green *et al.* (1991) because, with regard to anomalies of the fetus, this is very often not the case; termination of the pregnancy is the only option available in most instances. However, advances in intrauterine treatments, including surgery, are likely to be more widely available in the future, although many of these treatments are still in the experimental stages.

Sometimes the discovery of minor abnormalities, for example the extra digit, can create further problems. Some of these minor anomalies could indicate chromosome disorders and to determine whether or not this is the case might mean that the woman has to undergo further invasive procedures which could put the fetus further at risk. The final outcome could mean termination of the fetus and the minor anomaly could prove to be nothing of significance. Grant (1987) and Twining (1994) suggested that these new dilemmas are more trouble than they are worth for the pregnant woman, producing great anxieties which can be more harmful than helpful.

Women are often persuaded to have a scan in early pregnancy to establish or confirm the expected date of delivery, or they are persuaded in late pregnancy to have scans to monitor growth of the fetus and do not realize that viewing the fetus could reveal anomalies. The improved resolution of the machinery has led to an increase in the ability to diagnose fetal anomalies; anomalies that can become apparent at any stage of the pregnancy. Some structural abnormalities are visible from a very early gestational age and Nicolaides *et al.* (1994) have demonstrated that by measuring the nuchal fold of the fetus at 12 weeks' gestation the fetus at risk of suffering from Down's syndrome can be detected.

Another problem with screening procedures is that, by their very nature, they induce a certain level of anxiety in women. The offer of a screening test of any description immediately implies that there is an element of doubt about the health of the individual concerned (Shickle and Chadwick, 1994). Therefore, screening of the fetus produces a heightened level of anxiety for women. Green and her colleagues (Green, 1990; Green *et al.*, 1991) have examined the effects on women of scanning and maternal serum screening and have highlighted the importance of counselling women throughout the procedure. Marteau constantly argues that the psychological effects of prenatal screening have never been addressed (Marteau, 1989, 1990, 1993; Smith and Marteau, 1994). Hospitals providing counselling services to women who undergo ultrasound screening are very few. The technology has been introduced at such a rapid rate that provision of counselling is carried out on a very *ad hoc* basis, and usually in retrospect after a problem has been discovered. The lack of resources is often given as the excuse when health care providers are challenged.

Giving women the choice

Changing Childbirth (Department of Health, 1993) places the woman at the centre of her care. It opens with a chapter entitled 'Women Centred Care' and the key components include such statements as: 'Information about the local maternity services should be made readily available.' The recent document distributed to every household on the maternity services states categorically that women will have a choice whether or not to have a scan (Department of Health, 1994).

Choice concerning whether or not to undergo screening is of vital importance because of the possible implications of the results. However, this choice is often withheld because women are not given the relevant information (Proud, 1994, unpublished information). Green found that this lack of choice was a complaint many women voiced when undergoing prenatal screening; one woman was quoted as saying, 'It was my decision to have the termination and screening tests, but not the scan that was advised and booked for me. They made that decision; it was a mistake' (Statham and Green, 1993).

Informed choice is invalidated if the women do not have sufficient knowledge regarding the options available to them. However, it is not so easy to determine how much information to give so that an informed choice can be made. Wells (1986) has made several observations about the role of nurses in giving information to enable patients to make an informed choice. Nurses, he suggests, often act in a subservient role to doctors and are therefore liable to coerce patients into making decisions that accord with the doctors' wishes. Nurses can only give information if they have sufficient knowledge about the subject themselves. Emotional equilibrium is needed on the part of the nurse to express a rational informed opinion. The midwife's position is clearly defined in the Code of Professional Conduct which states, 'to prescribe or advise on the examinations necessary for the earliest possible diagnosis of pregnancies at risk' (UKCC, 1992). Whelton (1990) also considers the midwife's position and refers to the Code of Practice, which emphasizes the need to provide clients with up-to-date knowledge about all the tests available to them regardless of one's personal views. Niven (1992) has acknowledged the power midwives have in the giving of this information:

> The midwife who is preparing a patient for childbirth has considerable freedom to choose what, when and how to tell her many different aspects of parturition.... There are strong moral and ethical reasons why mothers and fathers to be, should be told about the risk of handicap in their baby, or about maternal risks, or about their baby's condition in utero.

There are some professionals who would argue that it is impossible to comply with these standards of information giving, primarily because the profession will always, and inevitably, have superior knowledge and possibly a bias when imparting the information. The woman and her partner cannot gain in a few minutes knowledge that has taken the professional years to obtain (Hamilton, 1983; Faulder, 1985; Katz, 1986; Whitfield, 1989). Holtzman *et al.* (1983) have argued that patients cannot make decisions when marred by situations of emotional instability or illness.

Faulder (1985) lists some very important points that concern the issue of consent. (See Chapter 1 for a full outline of the issues surrounding consent.)

(1) When the woman makes her choice it should be respected, even though some professionals might consider that the parents have not made the 'right' decision.
(2) A health professional can only advise the parents regarding medical matters; moral decisions, however, can only be made by the parents themselves.

Paternalism and safe practice

The health care professional views the scan as a screening process for fetal anomalies and an opportunity to create a basis or background from which to monitor a pregnancy. The offering of a routine scan in the first or second trimester of pregnancy can therefore be seen to be in the best interests of the woman. Women and their families usually enjoy their scan. This is often used to encourage women to have a scan and becomes part of the package of care that they are offered. This paternalistic attitude is often adopted because it is seen as part of good and safe practice. This can therefore override the woman's autonomy, the professional using their presumed superior and greater depth of knowledge to justify their action.

A lot of women expect this attitude from their carers. They have accepted it from their parents. They have been brought up to expect it from their doctors and even use it to their own advantage making comments like, 'My doctor says I must do such and such' (Gillon, 1991). McIntosh (1987) suggests that this attitude was particularly prevalent among the working class. In his study, he found women in Glasgow to be reluctant to make decisions regarding their care, happy to accept what was prescribed, believing it to be the best care possible. However, the medical profession and/or midwives have a duty to advise pregnant women on health or medical matters and this might conflict with the woman's own set of values and beliefs. To persuade a woman to make a decision which involves moral matters is not something the clinician should do; judgements of this nature must be left to the individual concerned. The professional's perspective of the best interests of the woman is not the only legitimate perspective (Chervenak and McCullough, 1991). As a result, what might be considered safe practice might not conform to what a woman decides (for example, the decision to refuse a scan) and the clinician should respect this.

Exactly why women accept the offer of a scan may have nothing to do with the reasons why it was offered (Green *et al.*, 1991). It is often accepted because women perceive it as a chance to see their baby on the screen. It is often seen as a social event, the highlight of a long pregnancy, when the partner and often the rest of the family are invited by the mother to attend. Several studies have indicated that it is a time when a positive relationship begins to develop between the mother and her baby (Campbell *et al.*, 1982; Reading and Cox, 1982; Reading and Platt, 1985; Reading *et al.*, 1988). Having a scan, therefore, can bring not only reassurance but also problems of its own. When they have a normal scan most women feel everything is all right, but an ultrasound scan can only detect a relatively limited number of abnormalities and subsequent events can occur in the pregnancy that might result in a less than satisfactory outcome (Green *et al.*, 1991), thus coming as a double shock to the woman who assumed that the findings of the scan had ruled this possibility out.

Regardless of whether women like their professionals to dictate or discuss their maternity care, they have a right to expect certain standards and quality of care. It would probably horrify women to realize, therefore, that very often the professionals performing their scan are not properly trained in the techniques. Midwives and obstetricians who perform ultrasound scans without proper training are abusing women's trust in their ability. One of the greatest dangers of ultrasound is the ease with which anyone can obtain a recognisable ultrasound image on the screen, thus lulling the operator into a false sense of security regarding their own expertise. The safety of ultrasound in pregnancy is a subject that has received a great deal of publicity and as yet no evidence of possible hazards have been found at diagnostic levels, but misuse is liable to result in unacceptable levels of ultrasound energy being used on pregnant women. Guidelines have been produced to avoid this (BMUS, 1989). Indiscriminate use by practitioners unskilled in its techniques and unaware of the potential problems of its misuse could result in unsafe practice. Little knowledge of the technique of scanning will also result in incorrect measurements and incorrect diagnoses of potential problems. This practice could result in doing the woman more harm than good.

The medical ethic of beneficence

The dictum that doctors should be beneficent goes back to Hippocrates in the 4th century BC and would seem to be an extremely simple ethic to adhere to but, as Thompson and Thompson (1987) acknowledge, in practice it can be very difficult. It can at times be hard to decide what is the good and caring thing to do and how to shield a woman from harm. The very fact of inviting women to partake of screening induces anxiety. Therefore, ways of reducing this anxiety should be a priority (Marteau, 1989, 1990, 1993). How much information should be given during and following a scan, especially when there is a suspicion of an abnormality, can also pose a dilemma for the professional. This includes another problem, is it always in the woman's best interests to tell the truth? This problem will be considered.

The importance of truth telling

Most mothers are aware when something is wrong. This has been described in several reports (Green et al., 1991; Proud, 1991) and nothing can take away the feelings of devastation that the diagnosis of fetal abnormality can bring (Green et al., 1991). A difficult situation often arises when there is a suspicion of an abnormality but, as is the case in many instances, no definite diagnosis can be given. The dilemma for the professional is how much, if any, information should be given to the woman. Medical practitioners are often accused of withholding information from patients especially if it is bad news, in the belief that it is in the patient's best interests (Donald, 1957). The giving of threatening information was evaluated by Greenwood (1973) and Kerrigan and colleagues (1993) who found that there seemed to be very little effect on the patient if they were told the truth when it was bad news, and the way doctors controlled the information was closely related to the way they handled their own emotions (Miyaji, 1993) rather than an attempt to protect the patient.

One argument against telling a mother the truth might be that the full situation is unknown. Another argument used is that the mother would not understand the situation or the implications if the truth were explained to her. A further reason put forward is that the woman would not want to know, especially if there is only a suspicion that something is wrong. Withholding information at this point might shield her from something that might never happen. The feeling of not wanting to frighten women unnecessarily is common. However, to deny women adequate knowledge and information fails to respect their autonomy and does not give them the correct information on which to base their decisions.

The woman's rights versus the professional's

It must not be forgotten that just as women have rights professionals also have rights and there are a number of situations where these rights can conflict. One of these relates to the revealing of the sex of the fetus. The natural response from most midwives would probably be that it is the mother's right to know, if it can be identified on the scan. However, consideration has to be given to other views which are often used to endorse hospital policies against revealing this information to the parents. One is that some women, particularly those wanting a child of a particular sex, will go to the length of obtaining an abortion if the expected baby is not of that sex. It is debatable whether or not the professional should become involved in such discussions. The moral question is one of whether the withholding of a fact is justified if the professional believes that the information they give will be used in a way that they cannot morally accept.

A further issue is the problem of visitors in the scan room. The scan is a screening or diagnostic procedure which needs to be undertaken in the shortest amount of time to obtain the maximum amount of information. This is part of good and safe practice (BMUS, 1989). There is no doubt that the presence of visitors in the scan room can, on some occasions, prolong the time of the scan but women often assert their right, as they see it, to bring visitors into the scan room, particularly partners. Sometimes these visitors can prove to be a distraction, especially if they hold the operator in lengthy conversation or if children are left to run around the department and are not kept under control by their parents. There can be an additional safety hazard if they interfere with the equipment. This is an unacceptable situation and one over which the professional should be allowed to exercise some autonomy (Gowland, 1992). Visitors can be welcome and they can share in the pleasure of seeing the baby on the screen for the first time. However, it can be difficult if an abnormality of the fetus is discovered, as it could inhibit any discussion taking place regarding the prognosis and the fetal outcome.

Conclusion

Professionals have a responsibility to provide the best quality of maternity care available by keeping themselves up-to-date with professional issues and not undertaking any procedures without having first received proper instruction. One of the biggest problems with ultrasound scanning is that it is so often abused, because it is easy to use and in most units very accessible and yet its potential is often not fully realized. Women have a right to be kept informed regarding every aspect of their care and good communication skills are therefore important. In order to provide good quality care adequate resources are necessary, not just up-to-date machinery, but staff with counselling skills and adequate knowledge of the latest technology so that they can assist women in making their decisions. Whether used to provide a diagnosis or as a screening tool, the scan should be an enjoyable experience for both the mother and her family, but this can only be assured if the ethical issues are addressed.

References

AIMS (1993). Ultrasound Unsound, *AIMS Quart. J.*, 5 (1), p. 24.

Bakketeig, L., Eik-Nes, S. H., Jacobsen, G. *et al.* (1984). Randomised controlled trial of ultrasonographic screening in pregnancy. *Lancet* (ii), 207–211.

Bennett, M. J., Little, G., Dewhurst, C. J. *et al.* (1982). Predictive value of ultrasound measurements in early pregnancy. A randomised controlled trial. *Br. J. Obstet. Gynaecol.*, 89, 338–341.

BMUS (1989). Prudent use of diagnostic ultrasound. Report of a working party. *BMUS Bull.*, 11–14.

Brock, D. J. H., Scrimgeour, J. B., Steven, J. (1978). Maternal alphafetoprotein screening for neural tube defects. *Br. J. Obstet. Gynaecol.*, 85, 575–581.

Bucher, N. and Schmidt, J. G. (1993). Does routine ultrasound scanning improve outcome in pregnancy: Meta analysis of various outcome measures. *Br. Med. J.*, **307**, 13–17.

Campbell, S., Reading, A. E., Cox, D. N. (1982). Short term psychological effect of early ultrasonic scanning in pregnancy. *J. Psychomat. Obstet. Gynaecol.*, **1**, 57–62.

Chervenak, F. A. and McCullough, L. B. (1991). Ethics an emerging subdiscipline of obstetric ultrasound and its relevance to the routine scan. *Ultrasound Obstet. Gynaec.*, **1**, 18–20.

Department of Health (1993). *Changing Childbirth. The Report of the Expert Maternity Group*, HMSO.

Department of Health (1994). *Maternity Services. The Patient's Charter.* HMSO.

Donald, M. (1957). *Medical Ethics: A Guide for Medical Practitioners.* Lloyd Luke.

Eik-Nes, S. H. (1984). Letter from Norway: Ultrasound screening in pregnancy. *Lancet*, **ii**, 347.

Ewigman, B. G., Crane, J., Frigoletto, F. *et al.* (1993). The RADIUS Study group. Effect of prenatal ultrasound screening on perinatal outcome. *N. Engl. J. Med.*, **329** (12), 821–827.

Giersson, R. T. (1991). Ultrasound instead of last menstrual period as the basis of gestational age assignment. *Ultrasound Obstet. Gynaec.*, **1**, 212–219.

Gowland, M. (1992). The case against visitors in the scan room. *BMUS Bull.*, **64**.

Grant, A. (1987). Cited in Pownall, M. Just a routine matter. *Nursing Times*, **83** (26), 19–20.

Green, J. M. (1990). *Calming or Harming.* Galton Institute.

Green, J. M., Strathan, H. and Snowden, C. (1991). Screening for fetal abnormalities: Attitudes and experiences. In *Benefits and Hazards of the New Obstetrics for the 1990s.* (T. Chard and M. Richards, eds), pp. 65–89. McKeith Press.

Greenwood, R. (1973). Should the patient be informed of innocent heart murmurs? *Clin. Paediatr.*, **12**, 468–477.

Grennert, L., Persson, P. H., Gennser, G. (1978). Benefits of ultrasound screening a pregnant population. *Acta Obstet. Gynaecol. Scand.* (Supplement) **78**, 5–14.

Hall, M. (1991). Health of pregnant women. *Br. Med. J.*, **303**, 460–2.

Hamilton, M. (1983). On informed consent. *Br. J. Psychiatry*, **143**, 416–418.

Holtzman, N. A., Faden, R. R., Chwalon, A. *et al.* (1983). Effect of informed consent on mother's knowledge of new-born screening. *Paediatrics*, **72** (6), 807–12.

Katz, J. (1986). *The Silent World of Doctor and Patient.* Free Press.

Kerrigan, D. D., Thevasagayam, R. S., Woods, T. O. *et al.* (1993). Who's afraid of informed consent? *Br. Med. J.*, **306**, 298–300.

Luck, C .A. (1992). Value of routine ultrasound scanning at 19 chase. A four year study of 8849 deliveries. *Br. Med. J.*, **304**, 1474–78.

McIntosh, J. (1987). Models of childbirth and social class: a study of 80 working class primigravidae. In *Midwives Research and Childbirth* (S. Robinson and & A. Thomson, eds). Chapman and Hall.

Marteau, T. (1989). Psychological costs of screening. *Br. Med. J.*, **299**, 527.

Marteau, T. (1990). Reducing the psychological costs. *Br. Med. J.*, **301**, 2126–2127.

Marteau, T. (1993). Psychological consequences of screening for Down's syndrome, still being given too little attention. *Br. Med. J.*, **307**, 146–147.

Miyaji, N. (1993). The power of compassion; Truth telling among American doctors in the care of dying patients. *Soc. Sci. Med.*, **3**, 249–264.

Neilson, J., Munjanja, S. P., Whitfield, C. R. (1984). Screening for small for date fetuses: A controlled trial. *Br. Med. J.*, **289**, 1179–1182.

Newham, J. P., Evans, S. F., Michael, C. A. *et al.* (1993). Effects of frequent ultrasound during pregnancy: randomised controlled trial. *Lancet*, **342**, 887–890.

Nicolaides, K., Brizot, M., Snijders, R. J. (1994). Fetal nuchal translucency: Ultrasound for fetal trisomy in the first trimester of pregnancy. *Br. J. Obstet. Gynaecol.*, **101**, 782–786.

Niven, C. (1992). *Psychological care for families.* Butterworth-Heinemann, pp. 134–49.

Persson, P. H., Grennert, L., Gennser G., *et al.* (1979). Improved outcome of twin pregnancies. *Acta Obstet. Gynaecol. Scand.*, **58**, 3–12.

Proud, J. (1991). The ultrasound scan: is it really necessary? *Modern Midwife*, **1** (2), 6–8.

Proud, J. (1994). Investigation into information giving prior to ultrasound scanning in pregnancy. Unpublished report.

Reading, A. E. and Cox, D. N. (1982). The effects of ultrasound examination on maternity anxiety levels. *J. Behav. Med.*, **5**, 237–247.

Reading, A. E. and Platt, L. D. (1985). Impact of fetal testing on maternal anxiety. *J. Reprod. Med.*, **30**, 907–910.

Reading, A. E., Cox, D. N. and Campbell, S. (1988). A controlled prospective evaluation of the acceptability of ultrasound prenatal care. *J. Psychomat. Obstet. Gynaecol.*, **8**, 191–198.

Robinson, J. and Beech, B. (1993). Ultrasound ??? Unsound. *AIMS Q. J.*, **5** (1) p. 8.

Salvesen, K. A., Vatten, L. J., Eik-Nes, S. H. *et al.* (1993). Routine ultrasonography *in utero* and subsequent handedness and neurological development. *Br. Med. J.*, **307**, 159–163.

Shickle, D. and Chadwick, R. (1994). The ethics of screening. Is 'screenitis' an incurable disease? *J. Med. Ethics*, **20**, 12–18.

Smith, D. and Marteau, T. (1994). Informed consent to undergo serum screening for Down's syndrome: the gap between policy and practice. *Br. Med. J.*, **309**, 776.

Statham, H. & Green, J. (1993). Serum screening for Down's syndrome: some women's experiences. *Br. Med. J.*, **307**, 174–176.

Thompson, J .E. & Thompson, H. (1987). Ethics and midwifery. *Midwifery* **3** (2), 75–82.

Twining, P. (1994). Routine obstetric ultrasound is more trouble than it's worth. *BMUS Bull.*, **2** (1), 34–35.

UKCC (1992). *Code of Professional Conduct*. HMSO.

Walkinshaw, S. (1992). Paper to Symposium on Issues in Fetal Medicine. Galton Institute.

Warsof, S., Pearce, M., Campbell, S. (1983). The present place of routine ultrasound screening. In *Clinics in Obstetric and Gynaecology. Recent Advances*. (S. Campbell, ed.) Vol. 10. No 3, W. B.Saunders.

Wells, R. (1986). The great conspiracy. *Nursing Times*, **21**, 22–25.

Whelton, J. (1990). Sharing the dilemmas. *Professional Nurse*, July, 514–518.

Whitfield, A. (1989). Informed consent: Does the doctrine benefit patients in the United Kingdom? In *Medicine and the Law* (A. Brahams, ed.) RCP Publications Ltd.

Chapter 5

Concepts of normality in maternity services: Applications and consequences

Soo Downe

It is not uncommon for midwives to pronounce themselves 'experts in normal childbirth'. This pronouncement goes largely unchallenged and is seen as a matter of some pride, even as a fundamental statement of identity. In using it, it is assumed that the term 'normality' does not need explanation. This chapter seeks to explore the meaning of the term and the consequences of its use. In the process it explores three applications of the concept of normality: in assessing the nature of pregnancy and birth; in deciding on the normality of the fetus; and in defining if the behaviour of the pregnant woman fits the norms of society. The definition of risk and applications of the concept will be examined and the implications for users of maternity services considered. The impact of technological screening on the ability to assess risk will be elucidated, and finally the implications of risk assessment decisions for the midwifery profession and its role in childbirth are highlighted.

Abnormality and risk

Normality is not a fixed concept, it is socially defined and changes over time. It was once perfectly normal to believe that the earth was flat and those who thought otherwise were blasphemers; that the body was controlled by humours; and that blood letting was good for the sick. Contemporary Western culture does not accept these concepts; indeed, for most people in the modern world, such ideas would be considered ludicrous. However, contemporary society is less willing to consider how quickly knowledge and knowledge bases have changed within the lifetimes of individuals, or to reflect on the possibility that some current firmly fixed beliefs will seem quaint in even half a century's time. In this ever-changing world, the definitions of normality are increasingly filtered through scientific and technological advances.

In terms of health in general, abnormality is becoming more often defined as a deviation from the average, with the potential for pathology, rather than as a pathological entity in its own right. The application of this shifting concept of 'risk of abnormality' in childbirth is having two major effects. First, and most importantly, it forces increasing numbers of women into widely defined risk groups on the grounds that a deviation from the average is an abnormality until proven otherwise. Second, it causes the practice of midwifery to be ever more narrowly circumscribed. These consequences are explored below.

Application of risk assessment

The concept of risk assessment has been a regular feature of care-giving, albeit implicitly, for many years: 'Implicit risk scoring has been in existence for millennia, and ... It has been embedded in the daily routine of clinicians for decades' (Alexander and Keirse, 1989). It is in the area of antenatal care that most effort has been focused, attempting prospectively to define the nature of risk. Many formal risk scoring systems utilize large databases of retrospective data and logistic regression techniques to identify women at risk. The idea is that if enough pieces of information about women are collected, and if enough is known about their outcomes in pregnancy and labour, predictions can be made about likely outcomes for other women with similar characteristics. Then, prophylactic intervention can reduce morbidity and mortality in these groups with the highest statistical risk. However, as Alexander and Keirse point out, there are many pitfalls with this type of data collection, not least in defining the relevant clinical data in the first place. Furthermore, the choice of abnormal outcome used in assessing risk is crucial. Often it is perinatal mortality. The problem with this measure is that, first, it is so rare that large numbers of women need to receive an intervention in order to decrease mortality by very small amounts, and second, the decrease may itself be due to a number of factors which are not amenable to manipulation by obstetric interventions.

The addition of weighted scales and cumulative scores only serves to compound these factors. The 1958 perinatal mortality survey and the consequent longitudinal National Child Development Study were probably some of the earliest sets of data used to assess risk (Butler et al., 1969). In 1970 the British Births Survey was published (Chamberlain et al., 1970). This proposed a scoring system for risk based on the 1958 data. The idea was that a cumulative score, which was weighted for the contribution of particular factors, would be a good predictor of outcome. The following comprised the antenatal prediction scoring system (and see Table 5.1). Risk status was defined as follows:

- 0–2: low
- 3–7: median
- 8 +: high.

Table 5.1 suggests that, all other things being equal, a woman having her second baby after a previous spontaneous abortion is at a fourfold greater risk of perinatal mortality in the current pregnancy than a woman who has not had a miscarriage. Given that fact that current predictions put the rate of miscarriage at between 10 and 15% (Bennett and Brown, 1993), this risk scoring alone would put many women into the median risk group. It must be acknowledged that at the time the data was collected, 1958, known miscarriages would probably have been at a later gestation than those currently diagnosed after very early pregnancy tests. However, the relative insensitivity of the scoring system cannot differentiate between an early and a late miscarriage, with their very different aetiology, and therefore its application (and the interventions that could be imposed as a result of its application) may not be appropriate for the individual. Spontaneous abortion due to a lethal dominant chromosomal abnormality may well be a good predictor of subsequent perinatal risk, but an unexplained loss at six weeks probably would not be.

Table 5.1 British Births Survey. Antenatal risk scoring system

Factor	Score
Maternal age	
20–29	0
<20 and 30–34	1
35 and older	2
Parity	
1 and 2	0
0 and 3	1
4 and over	2
Social class	
I and II	0
III	1
IV and V and unemployed	2
Unsupported mothers (single, separated, divorced, widowed)	2
Previous obstetric performance	
Stillbirth	4
Neonatal death	4
Abortion	4
Caesarean section	4
Medical history	
Hypertension (BP 140/90 or more before 20 weeks' gestation)	4
Diabetes	4

Effects on women

Risk systems are population-, not person-, specific; for example, in the British Births Survey (Chamberlain *et al.*, 1970), a 36-year-old social class one woman with no pre-existing disease, who had planned the pregnancy, who swam regularly and ate healthily, but who had one previous miscarriage at eight weeks, would score six and be in the median risk group. With her in that group would be a woman of the same age and class who had also had a miscarriage, but who smoked 40 cigarettes a day, often binge-drank, never took any exercise and whose pregnancy was completely unplanned, and unwanted. Further, as far as individual women are concerned, risk scoring is of no benefit if something cannot be done to modify the risk. In the case of events occurring before the current pregnancy (such as past obstetric history) or of present physiological data (such as maternal height), modifications cannot be made. Even though formal risk scoring is not often used now, informal assessment of risk is a part of everyday practice (see for example Hall, 1995), and its application is once again on the agenda following the exhortation in the government document *Changing Childbirth* (Department of Health, 1993) that purchasers and providers should: 'review the pattern of antenatal care in the light of current evidence.'

Such reviews imply risk assessment and the allocation of women into nominal risk groups. Handwerker (1994) discusses the ways in which the application of 'high risk' labels leads to the censoring of pregnant women who fail to comply with medical advice. The application of such risk markers, if pushed to their logical consequences, results in judging the abnormality, or even criminality, of women who are unable or unwilling to act on the scientific predictions (accurate or not) arising from them. This application of the concept of risk of the abnormal is an illustration of the potential imbalance between the attempt to effect benevolence for the baby while, at the same time, violating the principle of non-malevolence for the mother. Its most extreme consequences are court-ordered Caesarean sections against the will of pregnant women or even long-term imprisonment of drug-using women in pregnancy. These policies are based on an assumption that risk is the same as inevitable pathology and on a failure to assess the relative stressors and values of women and families in widely different cultures.

Cross-cultural assumptions also affect women's experience of the allocation of risk. The effect of maternal age is a case in point. The researchers analysing the National Child Development Study (Butler *et al.*, 1969) varied their categorization of age, but the most frequent allocation gave a low risk to women in the 20–29 years group, a median risk to those in the 30–34 years group and a high risk to the over 35 years group. This perception of risk obtains still today, although it is increasingly being questioned as the average age of child-bearing women creeps upwards. Recent researchers have demonstrated that, although intervention rates were universally higher in their sample of nulliparous women over 35 years old compared to younger matched controls, neonatal outcomes were not worse (Edge and Laros, 1993). This begs the question of cause and effect. Is the greater level of interventions found in older child-bearing women influencing the outcome positively, or are high intervention rates a function of the labelling of abnormality, with no improvement in the outcomes? As Edge and Laros point out, following a regression analysis of matched cases and controls, the higher Caesarean section rate amid the over-

35s was only partially explained by obvious complications. It may well be that, historically, older women were more at risk, either through grand multiparity, or because of poorly controlled underlying disease (such as diabetes) which caused subfertility and therefore delayed child-bearing. This underlying pathology is, however, less relevant in the late 20th century as more women choose to have babies later, fewer have large families and maternal disease is better controlled.

It is of interest, as an aside, to consider here current debate on the potential normality of post-menopausal women having babies. It could be argued that, in seeking to legitimize the contentious morals of such developments, their protagonists are seeking to underplay the previous concerns about maternal age. (See Chapter 10 for a consideration of the ethical implications of post-menopausal mothers.)

The uncertainty surrounding risk systems (and the potential for iatrogenic damage as a result of action taken in false-positive cases) is captured in the following comment from Golding and Peters (1988): 'If there is no valid preventative strategy—or if intervention itself carries a significant risk of hazard—then the whole process may be counter-productive, or even unethical.' This statement should be contrasted with that of Faragher (1988), who, in writing a chapter in the same book, states: 'Every item of information recorded at a booking visit has an association with risk.' Although recognizing that such an approach can lead to false negatives and false positives, he goes on to claim: 'False positives result in ... no detriment to the mother or baby who receive a level of attention greater than that actually required.'

This statement is arguable. It illustrates that, despite decades of interest, the perfect test has not been found, and that the iatrogenic risks of testing are still poorly understood and acknowledged. Despite our lack of understanding in the risk assessment area, we are now entering yet another new phase in the development of screening tests and consequent risking scores, that of the technological assessment, which is discussed below.

In summary, the benefits and iatrogenic drawbacks of risk-scoring are still to be established as Enkin et al. (1995) state:

> ... the potential benefits of risk scoring have been widely publicised, but the potential harm is rarely mentioned in the current literature. Such harm can result from unwarranted intrusion in women's private

lives, from superfluous interventions and treatments, from creating unnecessary stress and anxiety, and from allocation of scarce resources to areas where they are not needed.

Technological screening

The focus has now shifted from the retrospective analysis of risk in the general population to the discovery of physiological markers of variants in the individual. It may seem, as we gather increasing information about the microscopic changes in the body of a pregnant woman and that of her fetus, that we have at last obtained the skills and knowledge to understand fully the deviations from the normal and to begin to give women an individualized assessment of risk. However, it appears that even (and perhaps especially) in this field our knowledge is, at best, partial and its application contentious. The development of ever more powerful technology carries the potential to see what has not previously been seen, without the knowledge about its relative normality. When new markers are identified, it is not always clear whether they are merely non-suspicious variants seen only in a minority, or if they are true deviations. If the assumption is made that what is seen in the majority of cases is the normal, then what is seen in the minority of cases becomes the abnormal until proven otherwise.

Most researchers developing tests understand the necessity of maximum sensitivity (the ability to detect all the problems) and specificity (the ability to detect only the problems and to avoid the discovery of 'problems' where none in fact exist). Lilford *et al.* (1983), in discussing the value of the placental lactogen test in predicting the risk of fetal growth retardation, illustrate the point that what is normal and what is abnormal is, on occasion, a matter of debate and entails a trade-off between sensitivity and specificity for a particular marker or test: 'Clinical interpretation of any biochemical test depends on the definition of a cut-off point ... above or below which the patient is considered "abnormal" for the purposes of subsequent decision making.'

It could be argued that if a test is sensitive and specific, if it is testing for a problem that is of real concern to the individual as well as to society, and if there is a real chance of avoiding or eradicating the problem without causing harm that test passes, in an ethical sense, the rule of beneficence. However, tests should also pass the test of non-maleficence and it is here that the problem arises. If the above criteria are not satisfied, if a test does not pick up all those with the problem, or if it identifies some as having a problem when they do not, or if the problem is not seen as such by the individual or by society until the test makes it obvious, or if there is not a harm-free solution to the problem, one may begin to ask whether the test risks in itself becoming the cause of iatrogenic distress.

Sophisticated screening tests both reveal and define our experience of the abnormal. At the extreme, this concept encompasses the fetus itself. The relatively subjective decisions made when choosing the cut-off point for 'high risk' are particularly crucial in screening tests for fetal abnormality, where the chosen cut-off point has major psychological and physical implications for the woman, the fetus and their family. There is now a very large body of evidence relating to the use of tests and scans to identify the abnormal fetus, but very little literature on either the ethics of such definitions and their consequences, or on the dividing line between normality and abnormality in this context.

One of the key ethical problems at the heart of this explosion of screening and scanning is that the only cure for the supposedly abnormal child is the termination of the pregnancy (see Chapter 8). The psychological impact of this on parents and family, the potential malevolence, is as yet extremely poorly measured, let alone compared to the psychosocial consequences of parenting a child with profound disabilities. The ethical impact of the definition of abnormality in this area is as yet unexplored. How far will society go in assuming abnormality and in insisting on termination, or in refusing to support an abnormal child which the parents knowingly decide not to terminate? Will the elimination of the more obvious abnormalities render currently acceptable deviations from the average unacceptable in the future? Who decides what is abnormal when the prognosis for any individual fetus (even with a known chromosomal abnormality) is impossible to predict? It is important to note that even the development of such technology changes the experience of pregnancy itself for all women into one of potential abnormality, rather than anticipated normality (Rothman, 1994), and the impact of this revolution is yet to be assessed. Daker and Bobrow (1989) summarized this as:

Costs are not wholly financial, and it is equally important to weigh the human costs. Although screening programs may bring reassurance to some women who are tested, for others they may generate anxiety by merely raising the question of abnormality. The consequences of erroneous diagnoses must be a matter for particularly careful consideration.

Effects on midwifery practice

The marginalization of midwifery into the realm of the normal (as defined both by obstetricians and by midwives themselves) has taken place over the last century. The delivery of the breech baby serves as an example. Breech delivery has been redefined almost exclusively into the sphere of the obstetrician. In 1958, the *Myles Textbook for Midwives* (Myles, 1958) clearly locates breech presentation under malpresentation in the section entitled 'Abnormal labour' and states that a doctor should be informed if the breech persists beyond 32 weeks' gestation, mainly in order to attempt an external cephalic version. The potential complications arising from a breech delivery are noted, and the comment is made that:

> ... although midwives are permitted by the Central Midwives Board to undertake the delivery of breech presentations at home, they would be well advised only to do so in an emergency. The opinion of most obstetricians is that, because of the risks to the foetus, multiparae as well as primiparae should be delivered in hospital where expert assistance is available.

However, the textbook continues to assume that it will be the midwife who delivers the baby even in the complex delivery of the extended legs. It is also acknowledged that in even more difficult situations (such as extended arm or head) the midwife may be delivering the baby at home and that she therefore needs to be taught how to manage the situation. In this case, the abnormal is still seen to be within the domain of the midwife. Although textbooks being produced today (e.g. Bennett and Brown, 1993) continue to instruct midwives in the techniques of delivering the breech, it is increasingly uncommon for midwives to do so on their own responsibility, if at all. This fact is picked up by the midwives interviewed by Leap and Hunter (1993), in their analysis of the work of midwives and handywomen who began practising in the 1920s and 1930s. The authors state, 'although a breech birth at home would be considered an emergency nowadays,

Table 5.2 British Births Survey. Length of labour
risk score

Duration of labour	Score
Duration of first stage of labour:	
<12 hours	0
12–24 hours	1
24 hours +	2

in pre-NHS days such births were considered normal.' Edie B., one
of the midwives interviewed, said: 'Oh, I used to love delivering
breeches. The breech births were so easy. . . . And we never used to
have any problems with them.'

To assist a woman in a breech birth at home or in hospital was
by no means an unfamiliar activity to midwives until comparatively
recently; now it is seen as being inadvisable by most midwives. The
circular effect of changing obstetric practices on the diagnosis of
abnormality and the interventions caused by that diagnosis can
also be explored in this context. The 1970 British Births Survey
(Chamberlain *et al.*, 1970) proposed an intrapartum scoring system,
which scores length of labour as shown in Table 5.2.

This system is explained by the following statement: 'Duration of
first stage of labour—any factor which unduly prolongs labour may
constitute a risk of intrauterine hypoxia and infection; labour has
been rated as normal up to 12 hours, as of intermediate risk of 12–24
hours, and as a serious problem when extended beyond 24 hours. . . '
(Chamberlain *et al.*, 1970). It is interesting to ask how this rating
system is justified. Since length of labour is a factor midwives often
have to use in judging the normality or otherwise of labour, it is
worth exploring in some depth.

Berkeley *et al.* stated in 1931: 'Labour in primiparae lasts on average
about 15 to 20 hours. In multiparae, eight to ten hours can be taken
as the average time. . . . It is foolish to attempt to prophesy more than
approximately how long labour will last in any given case.' By 1958
Margaret Myles appears to be rather more certain and her statement
uses the language of normality as well as that of the average:

> . . . Seldom is the second stage less than an hour in a primipara and
> midwives are usually advised to consider 2 hours as being sufficiently
> long: the multiparous woman may have a second stage of 15 minutes
> or less and one hour is advocated as the limit of normal. The duration

of the third stage is between 10 and 20 minutes, and one hour is recommended as the limit of what could be considered normal. The consensus of opinion is that during the past twenty years the duration of labour has been shorter than previously, probably due to the greater use of relaxation and sedation. The figures below could be considered fairly average but experience proves that average figures can be misleading.

	First stage	Second stage	Third stage	Total
Primigravida	$12\frac{1}{2}$	2	$\frac{1}{2}$	15
Multipara	$8\frac{1}{2}$	1	$\frac{1}{2}$	10

A considerable number of primiparae have labours of under 12 hours, and by far the greater numbers of multiparae have labours of 6 to 8 hours and in many cases less than 6 hours.

Although the possibility of variation is accepted in the text, the only examples given are where labours are shorter than expected. This emphasis is reinforced in a subsequent textbook (Myles, 1975):

	First stage	Second stage	Third stage	Total
Primigravida	11	$\frac{3}{4}$	$\frac{1}{4}$	12
Multipara	$6\frac{1}{2}$	$\frac{1}{4}$	$\frac{1}{4}$	7

This later edition of Myles' text also states that the duration of labour has decreased in the last 20 years and adds oxytocin to the list of elements considered to have contributed to the change. Although authors of the most recent edition of the *Myles Textbook for Midwives* (Bennett and Brown, 1993) are careful not to impose limits, it is now almost impossible to ascertain the true limits of normally progressing labour within Western society because assumptions of risk associated with long labour have changed obstetric and midwifery practice to the point whereby labour has been redefined into preset time scales.

Effects on the midwifery profession

It can be argued that one of the factors influencing the change in perception of midwives about the sphere of their practice is that of midwifery regulation, and the consequent restriction of midwifery to an increasingly narrowly defined scope of practice. In pursuing this theory, it is of interest to note the historical arguments against the regulation of midwifery. As Donnison (1988) points out, many midwives practising prior to the 1902 Act were against legalization, feeling that it would bring them under the domination of the medical profession. This view is still current. Mason (1988), describing the debate about legalization of midwifery in Canada, comments on the opposition of some lay midwives to the change, on the grounds that it would restrict midwifery. She states: '. . . pressure mounted on the new almost-legal midwives not to deviate from fairly conservative standards of safe practice at home births.'

The counter argument now, as in 1902, rests on the need for legislation to ensure the maintenance of optimum practice or, more precisely, to allow for the censorship (and deregulation) of bad practitioners. This combination of push and resistance led to the creation of legislation that was based on restriction rather than enabling the midwife. The 1902 Midwives Act was 'an act to secure the better training of midwives, and to regulate their practice'. There is very little in the Act about training and a lot about regulation, including the setting up of the local supervision authority to 'investigate charges of malpractice, negligence, or misconduct' (Section 8(2)). The concept of such supervision implies that a line between a good and a bad practitioner will have to be drawn. This entails the establishment of parameters to safe practice. If there was good and consistent research defining such limits, and the negative outcomes that would result from transcending them, legalization describing them would be empowering for every midwife. However, this is still not the case and the regulation of midwifery, of necessity, limits some and restricts others.

When the 1902 Act was formulated, the concept of normality was not embedded within it. The Act did not mention the limits of midwifery practice or the appropriate time for referral. These were, however, outlined in detail in the 1903 rules (Towler and Bramall, 1986).

Although the rules no longer specify in detail what is to be regarded as abnormal, and therefore within the province of the doctor, lack of agreement remains between professions about where the line should be drawn between the normal and the abnormal and who should define that line. This is also an issue within midwifery itself. A study carried out by Ann Oakley and Susanne Houd (1990) illustrates this point. This included an examination of the nature of midwifery via interviews with 26 midwives and 21 obstetricians in a number of different European countries. The subjects were given specific case histories and asked for their opinion on what they would do in the circumstances (see Tables 5.3 and 5.4). They are of interest, because they reveal that there are not only differences between professionals in different countries, but also differences between professionals in the same country. However, what is most striking is the expectation of normal or of abnormal outcomes depends on the philosophy of the professionals in each case.

For example, the first UK midwife in Table 5.3 does not expect infection and so does not intervene. However, the Italian obstetrician in the same case has every certainty that infection will ensue and his aggressive management of the case is based on that expectation. In Table 5.4, the second Italian obstetrician is adamant that there is a risk of stillbirth and that is uppermost in the decision to induce. The UK midwife, however, while recognizing that others would act differently, does not judge the situation to be abnormal and thus does not actively intervene. These case histories indicate the different rules of abnormality operating for different practitioners, and their actions consequent upon these rules, even though the case history is the same.

Conclusion

The argument that the definition of the boundaries between normality and abnormality in maternity care is an essential element in understanding the position of midwifery in society is not new. However, the impact of new technologies on those definitions, and the relative position of power defined by them, is a new phenomenon in the taxonomy of normality and abnormality. William Ray Arney (1982), a sociologist, examined the phenomenon of the rise and dominance of obstetrics in Europe and America, differentiating three periods of development. First came the pre-professional period, characterized by a symbiosis between barber surgeons and midwives, with midwives dealing clearly with the normal, and barber surgeons

Table 5.3 Case study: Whether or not to intervene. (Reproduced with permission from Oakley and Houd (1990)). *Helpers in Childbirth: Midwifery Today*. Hemisphere Publishing Corp)

Case	Recommendations from care-givers (summarized)					
	Midwife, United Kingdom	Midwife, Italy	Midwife, United Kingdom	Midwife, Denmark	Obstetrician, Italy	Obstetrician, United Kingdom
A 30-year-old primipara goes into labour a few days past term. Labour starts with ruptured membranes at 6 p.m. At 8 p.m. she is in hospital. She is only dilated about 2 cm. Clear amnion, heart beat good. No contractions. What would you do from here?	I wouldn't have her in the hospital anyway. I'd just leave her, I wouldn't do an internal, no nothing. The danger of infection is very little at home anyway. So long as the amnion is clear, I'd let her wait several days	We wait 24 hours, but she must take antibiotics and see the doctor. After that we induce	I'd see if she has had any food, make sure she got her supper, and hope she gets a good night's sleep. If in the morning there hadn't been any action—if we'd done an internal, we would have tried to stir things up a bit—we might even consider an enema. I'd assume she'd want to avoid a drip; well, I would want to avoid a drip. I might encourage her to get up and walk around in the morning. Then after a few hours she'd have to have Syntocinon	I'd ask how she felt—if she was tired or if she was quite fit. I'd give her a massage and see if it caused any contractions. If by midnight she didn't have any, I'd let her sleep. We would have to induce her in the morning	If contractions haven't begun after 6 hours, I'd induce. If the first drip doesn't induce, I'd wait 6 hours and give a second. It's absolutely necessary to give antibiotics, and we must do a culture to make sure there aren't any pathological microbes in the vagina to begin with	I'd probably let her walk around for a while. They have a bath, and if they haven't had their bowels open that day, they get a course of suppositories. You don't normally give enemas, and you don't shave them either. I'd encourage her to walk about, and I'd feed her to give the uterus something to work on, and then I'd just wait and see what happens. If after 12 hours she hadn't done very much, then we'd offer her some Syntocinon. But again if they refuse (they don't usually refuse if you talk to them sensibly), the longer you leave them with the waters gone, the more risk there is to the baby

Table 5.4 Case study: induction (postterm). (Reproduced with permission from Oakley and Houd (1990). *Helpers in Childbirth: Midwifery Today*. Hemisphere Publishing Corp)

Case	Obstetrician, Italy	Obstetrician, Italy	Midwife, Greece	Midwife, Italy	Midwife, Denmark	Midwife, United Kingdom
				Recommendations from care-givers (summarized)		
A 28-year-old woman having her second baby is 12 days overdue according to dates and ultrasound. Baby's weight is estimated at 3600 g. Human placental lactogens and oestriol levels are normal. Hormone tests are OK. Her first child weighed 3500 g and was delivered at term +8 days. Her menstrual cycle is 4½–5 weeks. What should be done?	I'd wait until 42 weeks and then I'd do an induction. Meanwhile, I'd give her a kick chart and an amnioscopy every day. I don't take any notice of the menstrual cycle if I have 2 ultrasound scans	I wouldn't have let this pregnancy go over the due date by so many days. We'd have to do a series of tests to be sure the infant is mature first and then induce. After all, we're dealing with a case of potential stillbirth	As a midwife in Greece, I don't have the right to do anything in this case. I'd send the woman to the doctor, and he'll say what has to be done. I wouldn't induce labour. It's up to the doctor	If there's some dilatation of the cervix, I'd suggest an amnioscopy. If the amniotic fluid is clear, I'd wait 2 more days. Then I'd admit her to hospital so as to attempt oxytocic stimulation	First of all, I'd see how she felt psychologically and physically at this stage. Then I'd study her first pregnancy: time of delivery, if she was overdue then, too. Then I'd go back to the ultrasound and do a new calculation, remembering her long cycle. She'd be just about due now. I'd send her to the doctor next time because, according to our directives, she must see the doctor at 41 weeks	I'd check that she is well, still gaining weight, blood pressure normal, etc. I'd suggest that maybe making love might push things on a bit or even a dose of castor oil. She's not too much overdue, and it probably has something to do with her long menstrual cycle. A doctor at this stage would be more inclined to give a date for induction after doing an internal examination, but I'd be inclined to let the mother go longer and encourage the mother to do something herself

with the abnormal. The next phase, the so-called professional period, marginalizes the midwives, and perceives all births as having a pathological potential. He states that: 'The rational approach to childbirth which crossed the Channel into Britain undermined the symbolic basis of the traditional midwives' practice by blurring the demarcation between "normal and abnormal" births ... This reformulation of the ideological basis of midwifery was essential to the ultimate success of male midwives in their struggle against women practitioners (Arney, 1982). He goes on crucially to state that: 'The midwife had control ... over the distinction between normal and abnormal, and it was on the control of this distinction that her power rested.' He observes that the new theory of 'abnormality' did not have a clear application, but that it was enough to introduce the concepts, and to define the parameters, to effect the removal of power from midwives and essentially to cause the reallocation of the management of women whose bodies did not conform to a norm.

Arney proposes that currently a third phase of obstetrics exists, which he calls the monitoring period. He claims that this is characterized by a nominally team approach to maternity care, with the obstetrician in the role of 'expert', dealing with the physiological and the midwife allied with the women in the psychological sphere of care giving. The most interesting aspect of this analysis is the recognition that first, the technology needed for ever more precise monitoring is out of the control of the practitioners involved and second, that the extension of monitoring implies that it scrutinizes every aspect of the woman's life and makes a judgement on it. This aspect is particularly acute and the ethical problems particularly complex, when such scrutiny is deemed to put mother and child into conflict. The imprisoning of pregnant, drug-using women in some states of America, or the imposition of court-ordered Caesarean sections are the most extreme examples of the moral complexities that arise from the societal imposition of the concept of 'normality' on to individuals within that society. It is at this moral juncture that the development of ever more complex technologies for observing new and uninterpretable phenomena has its greatest potential for iatrogenic impact, both in terms of physical damage (when the true meaning of the findings are not known and intervention causes harm) and psychologically (when the general values of society conflict with the specific, even if unrecognized, values of the individual).

It may well be that the time has come for midwives to begin to recognize that the imposition of an abnormal risk status for women and babies is often not scientific and that, while in some cases it promotes benefit, in others it causes iatrogenic damage. If midwives are truly to be the experts in normality, they must also learn to defend the definitions of the normal, in order to protect mothers and babies and to promote optimum health gain. The role of lead professional in new forms of maternity care affords an excellent opportunity and a profound challenge to midwifery; for instance, can new technologies be applied sensitively and appropriately by expert midwives both to identify true pathology and to empower women in appropriate decision making, while at the same time preserving the normality of pregnancy and birth? This is the fundamental question for midwifery in the future.

Each one of us has the continuing and increasing responsibility to ask the question, 'Although we can do this, ought we to do it? The normal dimension is not a luxury that can be debated abstractly in some academic or religious cloister; it is a pragmatic imperative as we look forward to the 21st century' (James and Stirrat, 1988).

References

Alexander, S. and Keirse, M. J. N. C. (1989). Formal Risk Scoring. In *Effective Care in Pregnancy and Childbirth* (I. Chalmers, M. Enkin, and M. Keirse, eds). pp. 345–65, Oxford University Press.

Arney, W. R. (1982). *Power and the Profession of Obstetrics*. The University of Chicago Press.

Bennett, V. R. and Brown, L. K. (eds) (1993). *Myles Textbook for Midwives* (12th edition). Churchill Livingstone.

Berkeley, C., Fairbairn, J. S. and White, C. (1931). *Midwifery by Ten Teachers* (4th edition). Edward Arnold & Co.

Butler, N. R., Alberman, E. D. and Peel, J. (1969). *Perinatal Problems: the Second Report of the 1958 British Perinatal Mortality Survey*. E. & S. Livingstone Ltd.

Chamberlain, R., Chamberlain, G., Howett, B., *et al.* (1978). *British Births 1970*, vol. 2 *Obstetric Care*. William Heinemann Medical Books.

Daker, M. and Bobrow, M. (1989). Screening for genetic disease. In *A Guide to Effective Care in Pregnancy and Childbirth* (M. Enkin, M. Keirse and I. Chalmers, eds). Oxford University Press.

Department of Health (1993). *Changing Childbirth. The Report of the Expert Maternity Group*. HMSO.

Donnison, J. (1988). *Midwives and Medical Men: a History of the Struggle for the Control of Childbirth*. Historical Publications.

Edge, V. and Laros, R. K. Jr (1993). Pregnancy outcome in nulliparous women aged 35 and older. *Am. J. Obstet. Gynecol.*, **168** (6 pt 1), 1881–1885.

Enkin, M., Keirse, M. J. N. C., Renfrew, M. and Neilson, J. (1995). *A Guide to Effective Care in Pregnancy and Childbirth* (2nd edition). Oxford University Press.

Faragher, E. B. (1988). Practical approaches to data collection. In: *Pregnancy and Risk: the Basis for Rational Management* (D. K. James and G. M. Stirrat, eds), John Wiley and Sons.

Golding, J. and Peters, T. J. (1988). Quantifying risk in pregnancy. In: *Pregnancy and Risk: the Basis for Rational Management* (D. K. James and G. M. Stirrat, eds), John Wiley and Sons.

Hall, M. H. (1995) Antenatal care. In: *Turnbull's Obstetrics* (G. Chamberlain, ed.), Churchill Livingstone.

Handwerker, L. (1994). Medical risk: implicating poor pregnant women. *Soc. Sci. Med.*, **38** (5), 665–675.

James, D. K. and Stirrat, G. M. (eds). (1988). *Pregnancy and Risk: the Basis for Rational Management*. John Wiley and Sons.

Leap, N. and Hunter, B. (1993). *The Midwives Tale; an Oral History from Handywomen to Professional Midwife*. Scarlet Press.

Lilford, R. J., Obiekure, B. C. and Chard, T. (1983). Maternal levels of human placental lactogen in the prediction of fetal growth retardation: choosing a cut-off point between normal and abnormal. *Br. J. Obstet. Gynaecol.*, **90**, 511–515.

Mason, J. (1988). Midwifery in Canada. In *The Midwife Challenge* (S. Kitzinger, ed.), pp. 99–129, Pandora Press.

Myles, M. F. (1958). *A Textbook for Midwives* (3rd edition). E. & S. Livingstone Ltd.

Myles, M. F. (1975). *A Textbook for Midwives* (8th edition). Churchill Livingstone Ltd.

Oakley, A. and Houd, S. (1990). *Helpers in Childbirth: Midwifery Today*. WHO Regional Office for Europe, Hemisphere Publishing Corporation.

Rothman, B. K. (1994). *The Tentative Pregnancy: Amniocentesis and the Sexual Politics of Motherhood*. Pandora Press.

Towler, J. and Bramall, J. (1986). *Midwives in History and Society*. Croom Helm.

Chapter 6

Midwives and sexuality: Earth mother or coy maiden?

Catherine Williams

Introduction

In this chapter I explore the relationship between sexuality, the reproductive continuum, and the midwife. Initially, various personal experiences will be recounted that led me to suggest that the medicalization of childbirth has divorced sexuality from childbirth and has created the coy maiden midwife, at the expense of the earth mother midwife. These experiences are from my work as a health care worker in the late 1970s and early 1980s and also, more recently, from my work as a lecturer to student health professionals in higher education.

Having established that there does clearly seem to be a sexual component in the reproductive continuum, I suggest that the writing out or exclusion of sexuality in this context actually complicates, confuses and blurs the issues rather than making the sexual aspect safe. I suggest that all health professionals, particularly midwives, need to recognize and acknowledge the sexual nature of their work in order to be able to relate honestly to and support the person seeking their professional assistance.

Professional experiences

Looking back, the initial encounter that led me to question the relationship between sexuality and midwives was while I was doing a three-month obstetric course prior to starting my health visiting training. The specific incident was my first vaginal examination (VE). I can remember my response as if it were yesterday; I was stunned by how lovely her vagina was, how soft, warm, velvety and moist. I can remember saying, 'Oh isn't it lovely, so warm and soft? Isn't it a nice place to be? No wonder men like sex so much', as I gently explored the woman's vagina and tried to locate what the midwife was describing. The woman whom I was examining seemed to enjoy my enthusiasm and smiled, remaining relaxed. The midwife suggested that I should remove my fingers and that was enough. Nothing was said, but I was aware that I had transgressed one of those invisible rules that one meets occasionally in life. To put this in context, it was in the mid-1970s, women's consciousness raising had not happened yet in the North West of England, or if it had it had certainly passed me by. The Natural Childbirth movement was around but was very much a fringe activity and was disapproved of by most of the midwives I came across. At that time, I was not sure what rule I had transgressed but now I realize. To link the clinical VE with sex was a major sin. Not only that, but actually enjoying it and expressing my enjoyment of another woman's body was clearly a 'mortal' sin in the midwifery world. Childbirth was clearly divorced from sexuality, it was a medical not a sexual event.

Since then, having worked as a health visitor and then training and working as a midwife I have never, in the professional context, heard anyone mention how lovely a woman's vagina is or the possibility of a VE being enjoyable in any way. The emphasis has always been placed on the diagnostic function, one that is acknowledged to be very intrusive, may be uncomfortable and painful for the woman and rightly kept to the minimum in terms of frequency and duration. Recent discussion is even questioning its value both antenatally during labour and postnatally (Clement, 1994). Here I feel the need to make it clear that I was not getting a sexual buzz out of the situation but that I was acknowledging and enjoying the woman as a sexual being in the very sexual act of childbirth. It was very similar to the enjoyment and wonder I felt every time I was present at the spiritual and sexual moment of birth. Looking back at my midwifery experiences, I see that I learnt very quickly not to express or acknowledge the sexual aspect of childbirth at all; the sacred or spiritual was allowed outlet at times in response to particular women and their babies, but mostly it was all overridden by the medicalization of the whole event, everything was transformed into the clinical. Clinical with a humane side certainly, clinical with a 'natural' aspect too, but working in an NHS hospital this clinical perspective dominated.

I had always expected that the midwife would be the ultimate earth mother, a grounded sensual, sexy woman who was in touch with the rhythms of the seasons. To be socialized into a medicalized, coy, maiden midwife had been a real challenge to my assumptions. I would like to suggest a midwifery continuum with two images of the midwife at either end. At one end we have the earth mother, the grounded, raunchy, home-birthing midwife, who perceives childbirth not only as a life event but also as a sensual and sacred event. At this end of the midwifery continuum we have Ina May Gaskin saying: 'Every birth is holy, I think that a midwife must be religious, because the energy she is dealing with is Holy. She needs to know that other people's energy is sacred' (Gaskin, 1980).

Gaskin goes on to explain that by religion she means that, 'compassion must be a way of life' for the midwife. Another view of what I shall call the earth mother midwife is from Sheila Kitzinger (1991) who cites the Tao Te Ching's description: 'You are a midwife: you are assisting at someone else's birth. Do good without show or fuss. Facilitate what is happening rather than lead what you think ought to be happening. If you must take the lead, lead so that the mother is helped, yet still free and in charge. When the baby is born, the mother will rightly say: "We did it ourselves".' This earth mother midwife is 100% there for the birthing woman, endlessly giving, intuitive, sensitive, open, accepting, compassionate, loving, meeting her every need, truly holistic. A very wise woman.

At the other end of the continuum we have the medicalized midwife, the coy maiden, standing behind or beside the rest of the professional team within the masculine patriarchal obstetric system. Sheila Kitzinger starts one of her books (Kitzinger, 1991): 'In child birth today the obstetrician usually stands centre-stage. The midwife is invisible.'

This midwife may also be endlessly giving, kind, sensitive and aiming to meet the needs of the birthing woman, but she is also a product of her culture, the medical culture. She is endlessly connecting up the tubes and wires of technology and meeting the needs of the medical model. Not only has she (in England, at present) most probably been socialized into the nursing role, and all that entails, prior to becoming a midwife, but most of her midwifery socialization will be well within the medical model and she will be very fortunate if she has ever been present at a home birth.

I am not putting this midwife down, she may be, and probably is, a wonderful woman, but to stay in touch with the social, sexual and sacred aspects of childbirth in the sterile, aseptic, technical world of obstetrics is very hard. The midwives stand in coy uniforms that are reminiscent of the serving class, trying to meet the needs of very different groups of people, the pregnant women, the obstetrician's team and the hospital management structure. In these circumstances it is very difficult to become grounded enough to start to fight for the woman's needs and a fight is not a good starting point for her to reach her goal of being 'with' the birthing woman.

Most midwives in this country are probably somewhere along the continuum placed between the two extremes. My fear is that most are clustered towards the coy maiden end.

Three recent incidents, in particular, have led me to analyse further the relationship between midwives, childbirth and sexuality and I intend briefly to outline them prior to developing my discussion.

The first was during a fairly informal interprofessional meeting. We broke for coffee and I realized that I had started bleeding early and had no sanitary wear. I came back into the group and stated that I had started bleeding and asked if anyone had any tampons I could use. One of the midwives said, 'Oh yes' and disappeared out of the room. A few minutes later she came back in and came up to me and whispered that she had put, 'what I needed on top of the loo'. I felt I had been 'coy maiden midwifed'. I value the care, the concern and the thoughtfulness of her discretion, but it highlighted to me the 'coy maiden' approach to midwifery where discretion *can* become a barrier to naming what is, and concealing and silencing the reality and sexuality of women's reproduction. My bleeding is about being a woman, it is about my reproductive potential and it is about my sexuality. I do not want it concealed and made invisible as it so often is in our patriarchal society. This is often what we do to women who we meet in our jobs as midwives, we sanitize it, we create a discrete clinical barrier between us and most aspects of the reproductive continuum, from menstruation, through contraception, conception, assisted conception, antenatal interactions, childbirth and the postnatal period. This may well suit a lot of women who also view the process in a clinical way, but where is the sexual and the sacred for the women who do want to express their reproductive lives in this other way?

The second incident occurred whilst I was teaching about sexuality on the Midwifery Diploma. The students were mature and qualified nurses. We did an exercise that focused on their own bodies and their own sexuality. There was a lot of resistance and reluctance to address the issue of their own sexuality. It was more acceptable to address the sexuality of the 'other', the patient, and work with that but not to address their own. I also find this tendency with some of the student nurses I teach. In contrast, some other groups of students I teach, and do the same exercise with who have nothing to do with health professions, express much less resistance and engage in it enthusiastically. Interestingly, on the occasion of this second incident, during the lunch break after the exercise the student midwives started talking informally and when I returned they were wild. Barriers had dropped and the conversation was more like the end of a 'girls' night out' and the level of bawdiness makes Chaucer's *Canterbury Tales* seem polite! It reminded me of coffee break talk on the labour ward, especially on late or night shift. As one colleague said to me, 'Get a group of midwives together and it's all orgasms and penises'. So here we seem to have the 'coy maiden' operating in the formal context but in the informal context we perhaps see aspects of the 'earth mother'. Is it that the medicalized midwife is so repressed in the 'coy maiden' role but so much in constant touch with bodies and raw sexuality in her everyday work, that she needs some outlet and once this is provided, out it pours? Would it not be better for sexuality to be an acknowledged part of the midwife–patient relationship?

The third incident again involves my teaching role and my increasing awareness of the complications in the lives of the students. When I teach subjects such as domestic and sexual violence, the amount of students who have experienced abuse is significant. This undoubtedly reflects the increasing awareness and incidence of child sexual abuse and rape in our society at large (Scully, 1990; Tidy, 1994), so is not surprising in itself. However, it does have implications for the health professions, particularly midwifery, because the focus is on the sexual event of reproduction. Certain sessions have aroused deep pain for some of the women students and I feel particular concern about whether they can help others if they are not healed themselves.

So where does sexuality come into all this? The two main discourses Tess Cosslett has identified (1994), the 'natural' and the 'medical', will be employed to look at what role sexuality plays. I will then discuss what the implications are for the midwife and the midwife–client relationship if we do not acknowledge the reproductive continuum as a sexual process.

Where does sexuality come into all this?

Birth is the biological end result of heterosexual intercourse, on the occasions that conception takes place, so on this biological level we can fairly assuredly assert that childbirth is a sexual event. However, with the increasing development of contraception, the gap between heterosexual intercourse and conception has been steadily widening. Add to this the developments in assisted conception and the two become even further apart; conception itself becomes a clinical event and sometimes even a scientific laboratory event.

Tess Cosslett (1994) suggests that there are three discourses of motherhood: the natural, the medical and the old wives' tales. The two images of the midwife that I am using in this chapter, the coy hand maiden and the earth mother, neatly fit into two of the main discourses.

Additionally, sexuality is more than heterosexual intercourse, though this is sometimes difficult to perceive in late 20th century English culture and, rather than get into a long discussion on the cultural construction of sexuality, I would simply like to quote from the book *Our Bodies Ourselves* (Phillips and Rakusen, 1979):

> Sexuality is much more than intercourse. It is a pleasure we want to give and receive. It is a vital expression of attachment to other human beings. It is communication that is fun, playful, serious and passionate ... sexual feelings and responses are a central expression of our emotional, spiritual, physical selves. Sexual feelings involve our whole bodies.

Natural childbirth discourse and the earth mother midwife

In England Sheila Kitzinger is probably the most well known natural childbirth proponent and educator. She argues that childbirth is, 'part of a woman's whole psychosexual life—not simply ... an isolated occurrence at one end of her body' (Kitzinger, 1979).

Some of the women from the 'Farm Community in Tennessee' write about their experiences in Gaskin's book *Spiritual Midwifery* (Gaskin, 1980). I quote some of them to illustrate the sexual nature of their experience of childbirth. 'The rushes (contractions) started to turn me on. It feels like William (her partner) and I learned how to kiss each other in a heavier way than we'd been into before.'

Karen also talked of her labour in similar vein:

> My rushes hardly felt heavy at all, but I knew they must be because I was opening up. We just kept making out and rubbing each other. We got to places that we had forgotten we could get to. Since that day we have been remembering to really get it on. Going through the birthing I felt his love very strong. It was like getting married all over again.

Another woman, Cara, who trained to be a midwife at the Farm says: 'Over and over again I've seen the best way to get a baby out is by cuddling and smooching with your husband. That loving sexy vibe is what puts the baby in there and it's what gets it out, too' (Gaskin, 1980).

Kathryn Rabuzzi (1994) suggests there is a growing body of accounts of childbirth that not only acknowledges, but celebrates, the sexual aspect. Marilyn Moran's research (cited in Rabuzzi, 1994) into home birthing gives another insight into the erotic aspect of childbirth.

> I dreamt of John holding me tenderly during labour and after the baby was born—like RIGHT after. Naturally this happened! It was a natural response to the love and the sexual aspect of birth.

A husband of another woman having a home birth said:

> The birth was not only painless, but very pleasurable. We had never read about this aspect, and it took us both by surprise. As the baby crowned, I knew from Jean's look and sounds that she was having an explosive orgasm, which rolled on and on. What a long way from the pain and agony of conventional myth.

So there is clearly much evidence from heterosexual women, their partners and their midwives in the natural birth movement to support the suggestion that childbirth is a sexual event.

Likewise women have described pregnancy as being a very sexual and erotic time for them. Phyllis Chesler (cited in Rabuzzi, 1994) addresses her unborn child:

> I want to have orgasms without foreplay three or four times every day.
> I look at your father slyly, passively. I insist he come back to bed,

'now'. If we're outside, I suggest we borrow a friend's bedroom, or sneak into a hotel restroom, 'just for a minute'.

I am without shame. Never have I been in such sexual heat. Is this natural in pregnancy? Or am I enjoying my lust because I think it unnatural, taboo? What exactly is so arousing, so pleasurably 'lewd' to me about a woman with a round, fat belly initiating orgasms in Mediterranean heat? Is my body remembering something? Can bodies do this? . . . During and after love-making I watch my stomach, I watch you, like a voyeur, as if I'm not present. There's a direct line from my *consciousness* of your existence to my clitoris. Watching my belly, having my belly seen by another, seems to throb this mysterious line awake.

My serpent rises lazily, a full four feet, then coils back into its clitoral hood. My tiger is gone, my tiger returns, restless, ready to prowl again.

This delicious quote says it all and contrasts strongly with my experience as a midwife in the medical model when women frequently asked whether it was all right to have sexual intercourse with their partner and whether it would harm the baby. It was as though they had lost their power to decide and feel what was right for themselves.

Rabuzzi (1994) also suggests the possibility of an erotic relationship between the woman and the fetus. They are united as one and once the woman actually feels movements she can feel another being inside her and as Rabuzzi says this, 'opens up a whole new dimension of sexual experience.' She questions whether there is a closer relationship and suggests that from quickening to birth, 'the two relate as romance promises all lovers do. This is the bliss every lover craves.'

Clearly natural childbirth has a lot to say about the sexual experience of pregnancy and childbirth and there is also much evidence (Stanway and Stanway, 1978; Gaskin, 1980; Rabuzzi, 1994) to support the connection between sexuality and breast feeding. The midwife clearly needs to be an 'earth mother' to facilitate these women's experiences.

Medical discourse and the coy maiden midwife

In great contrast to the natural childbirth discourse, medical discourse, Tess Cosslett (1994) suggests, is that of male technological and scientific procedures taking childbirth out of the hands of women and setting it in the context of the powerful, male-dominated institution of the hospital, whereas the natural childbirth context seemed to be focused very much on the home birth and the power of the woman.

So where does sexuality fit into the context of pregnancy and childbirth in the medical environment? Rabuzzi (1994) cites a male obstetrician's observations:

> For years, convinced of the fact that delivery of the head constituted, owing to the perineal distension, the most painful phase of childbirth, we traditionally administered an anaesthetic to the parturient. It is striking to observe that women who have been conditioned by the psychoprophylactic method frequently declare that delivery of the head affords them the most exhilarating moment of the entire event. Indeed, we have frequently observed that the birth of the head, far from producing the usual tearing pain, stimulates an intense thrill, very close to that of orgasm.

It is interesting that he links the sexual experience of childbirth to women who have trained in psychoprophylaxis and therefore likely to have links with the natural childbirth movement. Rabuzzi clearly sees this obstetrician as an exception and suggests that patriarchal culture has such a block against seeing any potential for the erotic in childbirth that all the sensations are conventionally labelled pain or discomfort.

I remember while working on a postnatal ward a woman asking me for an early discharge. Her answer to my enquiry as to the reason was that she felt so sexual after the whole experience of childbirth and breast feeding that she wanted to get back to her partner as quickly as possible. Clearly, some women can find the experience sexual in the medical setting.

However, as many of us know, sexuality is not all bliss, orgasms and the earth moving. It can also be about miscommunication, misinterpretation, pressure, powerlessness, feeling empty, fear, failure, abuse and violence to name a few. Kitzinger (1992) has written about how for many women childbirth can become an 'ordeal in which they are disempowered.' She compares the language these women use to describe childbirth to the language used when describing experiences of sexual violence. Kitzinger clearly points out that this is not an experience only to be found in hospital but that women were also writing of horrific experiences of childbirth at home 40 years ago. But with the increase in technology, intervention and a medicalized and hospitalized childbirth the opportunity for intervention has increased. Many of the women writing to Kitzinger had been subjected to a technological childbirth and they used words such as 'rape', 'assault', 'abuse' and 'violence' in the description of their childbirth experience.

Kitzinger (1992) suggests that the theme of powerlessness is common to the women and goes on to show the clear similarities between powerless childbirth and rape: from the physical pain and damage, the lack of personal identity, to the emotional blackmail that can be used to ensure the patient or victim goes along with it. 'In childbirth, as in rape, a woman may be stripped, forcibly exposed, her legs splayed and tethered and her sexual organs put on display to all comers.'

She goes on to say that when women describe it they use the 'language of pornography' (Kitzinger, 1992). The women often blame themselves, and again, as in rape, the professionals involved often reinforce this. Kitzinger clearly shows the similarities of the women who feel they have been violated by the obstetric management of their labour and women who have been raped. The connection between childbirth and sexuality is all too clear in her analysis of these women's accounts. She concludes: 'Rape is endemic in our society. The western way of birth proves often to be another form of institutionalized violence against women.'

So where is the earth mother and the coy maiden?

Indeed, where is the midwife in all this? In Kitzinger's chapter discussed above (Kitzinger, 1992) there is only occasional mention of the midwife. She focuses on technological intervention and male violence at an institutional level as an explanation. Rabuzzi, from the USA, focuses on the male patriarchal obstetrician when considering the medical model. When discussing what she calls the 'midwifery model' (Rabuzzi, 1994) she focuses very much on midwives like Gaskin whose emphasis is on a spiritual and community experience in the home environment, very much the earth mother image of the midwife. In fact the midwife gets off very lightly in many current critiques of the process of child bearing. I wonder if this is justified. Where are the midwives during these labours where women feel abused and raped? Are they coy maidens standing by the side of the woman, being 'with' the woman but also being endlessly discreet and caring, not seeing the situation as abusive because it is shrouded in the clinical medical terminology of 'being in the patient's interests?' Are they so co-opted into the male medical system that they see the situation through the male medical gaze rather than from a gynocentric view? Do they not see it because childbirth is a medical event and not a sexual event? If they perceived the whole process as a sexual event that is important in women's lives would that change things? Could it alter their perception?

Muriel O'Driscoll (1994) has presented some brief case studies, one of which was of a woman who refused to be examined by the doctor antenatally. It was the midwife who explained the reasons for the examination and despite the woman's fear it was done. The woman had been gang-raped as a teenager and could not tell the midwife as, 'she (the midwife) was very busy.' O'Driscoll states that: 'Sometimes the midwife is a prime player but not always to good effect.' I think it is important to recognize the midwife's role in these situations; she must not be the doctor's hand maiden standing on the side lines, reinforcing the status quo.

Helen Tidy (1994) also graphically illustrates in her case study how going through childbirth can bring back hidden memories of child abuse. I quote at length as this woman's experience makes such a clear point:

> ... she coped well throughout the first stage, but the change to the second stage caused her to panic as she felt the baby descend through her pelvis. The similarity between an adult penis being forced inside the body of an 8-year-old and a fetus descending through the birth canal must be striking (Rose, 1992). When she shouted for help, the midwife used the exact words her abuser had used, 'Shh—don't cry!' reinforcing her feeling of abuse.

O'Driscoll (1994) sympathetically discusses the role of the midwife in relation to childbirth and sexuality, suggesting that they need to 'explore their own reactions' to vaginal examinations and that they need to 'remember that touch, pain and physical examinations can unlock hidden terrors.' She suggests a feminist approach, encouraging a midwife to be assertive and to act as an advocate for the woman. This is moving from coy maiden midwife further down the midwifery continuum towards the earth mother.

I would go further and suggest that not only do midwives need to look at their own feelings about VEs but they need thoroughly to explore their own issues around sexuality and then apply this understanding to the process and interactions around child bearing in our culture. I suggest that all midwifery education, including and especially refresher courses, should have space for initiating and developing this sexual awareness of midwives; hopefully this in turn will enable them in Jenny Kitzinger's words to, 'ensure that the care they offer counteracts rather than re-enacts the violation of women's bodies' (Kitzinger, 1993).

The coy maiden midwife often appears to me as without awareness of her sexuality. Yes, she may be very 'sexy' as male defined but she has not got in touch with her own female definition of what is sexual. I think this is socialized out of the midwife during both her nurse and midwifery education. Sexuality, although now much discussed and talked about, is somehow paradoxically still a very private area, full of taboos.

In the medical model, sexuality is mostly medicalized in order, perhaps, to control it and make it safe. Modern obstetric relations reproduce the perceived heterosexual norm of our society; the male obstetrician in charge and in control of women's bodies and the women complying, on the whole. With this clinical attitude and environment, discretion and professional distancing put up barriers to the dangerous sexual element and hence this is controlled and made safe.

But safe for whom? Certainly not safe for the women who write about their experiences to Sheila Kitzinger in terms of 'rape', 'violence' and 'abuse', nor the others who seek or do not seek help for problems following childbirth that O'Driscoll has highlighted. Is the medicalization of childbirth actually trying to create safety from women's sexuality and the sacred power of women's creativity? Rabuzzi (1994) explores how through mythology the sacred act of creativity has been taken from women and given to men. She suggests that since men do not have this natural means of connecting to the sacred, they need to create it in their culture and diminish women's natural connection to the sacred through controlling childbirth. Is today's obstetrician the modern-day equivalent of Zeus giving birth to Dionysus? In a patriarchal society the male needs to be in control, have power over, and, even more importantly, have a role in reproduction and creativity.

Perhaps the male medicalization of reproduction also controls women's sexual relations around childbirth by reasserting the heterosexual norm of male power and control. In a more gynocentric approach to childbirth, where the sexual and sacred element of childbirth was recognized as part of the process, the relationship between the birthing woman and the midwife could be a lot more intimate and intense. Rabuzzi (1994), discussing a midwifery model of labour and delivery, points out that these midwives see their role as a holistic process:

> A key word in this process is community—the community to which the childbearing woman belongs and the community that the midwife creates with her, for the relationship that develops between a labouring woman and her birth attendant is often astonishingly close . . . it can also create community at a very deep level.

She reinforces this picture by quoting Michel Odent's observations of the midwife at work: 'Body to body, skin to skin, a midwife will rely on touching and holding a woman, rather than speaking to her' (Rabuzzi, 1994).

Both Odent and Kathryn Rabuzzi talk of the relationship as 'communion'. 'Communion at its holiest, this sharing of the creating of new life clearly manifests the sacred dimension of childbearing.' It also clearly demonstrates the sexual dimension of the relationship. This intimate intense woman-to-woman relationship clearly challenges the perceived norm of heterosexuality. Perhaps homophobia and, in particular, the fear of women's close relationships is another factor behind the male medicalization of reproduction and the creation of barriers between professional and patient. If the midwife has not explored her own attitudes, ideas, assumptions and prejudices around sexuality this may seriously affect her interaction and relationships in her occupation. She may assume the woman is heterosexual which may lead her to give inappropriate advice, i.e. suggest contraception or ask inappropriate questions about the father of the baby. Presumption of a heterosexual lifestyle can lead the woman to feel very undermined (Rose and Platzer, 1993). With lesbophobia so common in nursing (Eliason and Randall, 1991), we may presume it to be similar in midwifery. Donna Tash and Janet Kenney (1993) cite an American study where lesbians described 'ostracism, invasive personal questions, shock, embarrassment, unfriendliness, pity, condescension and fear from health caregivers.' Not exactly 'the body to body, skin to skin' experience that I cited earlier. Lesbophobia may cause the midwife to withdraw from this intimate, intense woman-to-woman relationship.

The wounded healer

If we add to this quagmire of complex human relationships the midwives I have already mentioned earlier, who are themselves victims of child and adult sexual abuse, the situation becomes even more difficult. If the midwife herself has been abused and has not worked it through and is with a woman in labour who is going through an experience which she describes later as, 'I feel invaded and mutilated ... I don't feel the same person any more' (Kitzinger, 1992), it is no wonder that she cannot speak up, cannot defend the woman and cannot be the woman's advocate.

I come back to my point about midwifery education and the essential inclusion of sexuality within preregistration and postregistration courses. I would also suggest this area of education for *all* other health professional education (and I include doctors under this heading), but argue that for midwives it is even more important due to the sexual and intimate nature of their work. It is important for the woman who has been sexually abused to work through her experience, come to some understanding of it and with help lay some of the trauma to one side, so that she can be more comfortable with her own sexuality and thereby, hopefully, be more comfortable with other people's when she is working in a healing capacity. It is very difficult to heal someone else's wound when one's own wounds are bleeding profoundly and are intensely painful. We need to heal our own wounds before we attempt to heal others.

Conclusion

> 'Woman's sexuality represents the interface between two of the most potent and insidious forms of oppression—gender and sexuality' (Gordon and Kanstrup, 1992).

We need to move the pregnant woman centre stage, closely accompanied by the midwife and diminish the power and influence of the medical model and the obstetrician. The woman-centred care advocated in *Changing Childbirth* (Department of Health, 1993) sets the scene for this to happen. This, combined with recent changes in midwifery education, such as increasing the numbers of centres that now provide direct entry to midwifery and more midwives moving into higher education, opens doors to change. Through education midwives can be taught to examine and challenge the status quo. They can be encouraged to address the issues of sexuality and move away from the coy maiden towards the earth mother. Not in any way to impose this on women, the last thing we want is for the pregnant woman to feel that she 'ought' to experience it sexually as some women do in natural childbirth, but we need to recognize the diversity of women's needs and the complexity of the sexual aspect of the reproductive continuum in order to enable women to do what they need to do and the midwife to support her in whatever choice the woman makes. So to paraphrase O'Driscoll's (1994) quote I used earlier, we need the midwife to be the prime player in the professional team but *always* to *good* effect. Thus, it becomes an ethical imperative to make sure that midwifery practice is guided by the principle of beneficence and what the exercising of this principle means in practice must be based on a deeper understanding of women's experiences of childbirth.

Ignoring sexuality or allowing it to be subsumed under the medical model into a clinical event rather than a sexual life event is rather like trying to plug a volcano with liquid cement; we will all get splattered eventually. We need to acknowledge that a sexual relationship is present in our professional relationships. Failure to recognize this as midwives means that we restrict women's needs for both sexual privacy and for sexual expression.

References

Clement, S. (1994). Unwanted vaginal examinations. *Br. J. Midwifery*, 2, 368–370.

Cosslett, T. (1994). *Women Writing Childbirth: Modern Discourses of Motherhood*. Manchester University Press.

Department of Health (1993). *Changing Childbirth. The Report of the Expert Maternity Group*. HMSO.

Eliason, M. J. and Randall, C. E. (1991). Lesbian phobia in nursing students. *West. J. Nurs. Res.*, 13, 363–374.

Gaskin, I. M. (1980). *Spiritual Midwifery*. The Book Publishing Co.

Gordon, G. and Kanstrup, C. (1992). Sexuality—The missing link in women's health. *ids Bull.*, 23, 29–37.

Kitzinger, J. (1993). Counteracting, not re-enacting, the violation of women's bodies: The challenge for perinatal caregivers. *Birth*, 19, 219–220.

Kitzinger, S. (1979). *Education and Counselling for Childbirth*. Schocken Books.

Kitzinger, S. (1991). *The Midwife Challenge*. Pandora Press.

Kitzinger, S. (1992). Birth and violence against women. Generating hypotheses from women's accounts of unhappiness after childbirth. In *Women's Health Matters* (H. Roberts, ed.), Routledge, pp. 63–80.

O'Driscoll, M. (1994). Midwives, childbirth and sexuality. *Br. J. Midwifery*, **2** (1), 39–41.

Phillips, A. and Rakusen, J. (1979). *Our Bodies Ourselves*. Penguin Books.

Rabuzzi, K. A. (1994). *Mother with Child*. Indiana University Press.

Roberts, H. (1992). *Women's Health Matters*. Routledge.

Rose, P. and Platzer, H. (1993). Confronting prejudice. *Nursing Times*, **89** (31), 52–54.

Scully, D. (1990). *Understanding Sexual Violence*. Unwin Hyman.

Stanway, P. and Stanway, A. (1978). *Breast is Best*. Pan.

Tash, D. T. and Kenney, J. W. (1993) The lesbian childbearing couple: A case report. *Birth*, **20**, 36–40.

Tidy, H. (1994). Effects of child sexual abuse on the experience of childbirth. *Br. J. Midwifery*, **2**, 387–9.

Part Two

Technological Issues

Chapter 7

Ethical issues in neonatal intensive care

Pam Miller

Introduction

Few people with any interest in the subject can be unaware of the immense changes that have taken place in neonatal intensive care over the last few years. Treatment is offered to ever smaller and more immature babies. Equipment for measuring every conceivable parameter is constantly refined and most vital functions can now be sustained, for some time at least, by some form of machinery.

However, it has fittingly been said that, 'The machinery in an intensive care unit is more sophisticated than the codes of law and ethics governing its use' (Lee and Morgan, 1989). Those who work in neonatal intensive care units usually do so because they enjoy combining the care of babies with developing technological skills. These skills have to be augmented by an understanding of the ethical questions that might arise in this environment. This chapter will attempt to consider some of the ethical issues that confront nurses and midwives working in neonatal intensive care units, addressing such questions as: should all babies born alive be offered intensive care regardless of gestation; what should be the criteria for withdrawing intensive care; how should dying babies and those born with congenital abnormalities be managed, and finally, how should scarce resources best be used?

Approaches to decision-making

Initially it may be helpful to look at some of the beliefs that influence decision-makers in the neonatal field. James Walters, a philosopher, describes (Walters, 1988) four recognized decision-making approaches and it is likely that those involved in making ethical decisions base their decisions on one or more of these positions, even if they could not define it so exactly. Walters' four approaches are as follows.

(1) Value of life: this is the principle that every life is sacred and that factors such as quality of life and the cost of treatment have no bearing. This principle is most strongly developed in the Judaeo–Christian belief that man is created in the image of God, but it is also affirmed by most other major world religions (Whyte, 1989). One of the possible consequences of denying this principle was seen in the philosophy of the Nazi party in the 1930s which deemed some lives were 'not worthy to be lived' (Ramsey, 1982). Ignoring the intrinsic value of human life may also undermine the public's faith in the medical profession. However, most of those who adhere to this belief would admit the relevance of 'quality of life' considerations when making decisions about a baby's treatment.

(2) Parental authority: this approach sees the parents as the rightful decision-makers for an infant who is unable to make its own decisions. Since parents are responsible for most of the decisions about their child's upbringing while he or she is a minor, it is inconsistent to deny them this right in the neonatal period. They will also have to bear the brunt of the care if the child is handicapped. However, during the emotionally fraught time after the birth of a very immature or abnormal baby the parents may not be in a fit state to make crucial decisions, nor will they necessarily be able to grasp the degree of handicap anticipated and what that might mean for the child. It is also debatable whether a parent should feel that the responsibility for their child's life or death rests solely with them.

(3) Best interests: here the baby's best interests are seen as the criteria on which to base decision-making and treatment should result in a 'net benefit' to the infant. Although a high value is put on the infant's life, this approach recognizes that aggressive intervention will not always be in the child's perceived best interests. However this approach, although basically rooted in common sense, is of

limited use because it is difficult for anyone to be certain what the baby's best interests are, both because the prognosis is often uncertain and because no one can know what the child, if in a position to do so, would choose.

(4) Personhood: this is a concept in direct contrast to the belief in the sanctity of life which claims that only the possession of certain capabilities, such as self-consciousness, the ability to reason and to suffer and a sense of the future, confer personhood and therefore the right to life. As neither the fetus nor neonate possesses these capabilities, they have no automatic right to life. Proponents of this view, for example Kuhse and Singer (1985), qualify their position by reasoning that even though a neonate has no intrinsic right to life, if the child is wanted by its parents or by adoptive parents, it would be wronging them to kill it. This approach is at such variance with the deeply felt belief in the sanctity of life that it is unlikely to gain much credence among staff and parents in neonatal units in countries with a basically Christian heritage such as Britain (Walters, 1988).

Walters acknowledges that all these approaches are in some way unsatisfactory in providing a formula for settling hard questions and goes on to suggest a further approach, which he calls 'proximate personhood'. The central contention of this approach is that all newborns whose lives approximate personhood should receive at least ordinary treatment (Walters, 1988). Approximation to personhood concerns the state of the child at birth and the potential for development. If a normal newborn baby, or a baby with minor abnormalities, has reasonable potential to develop the capabilities of personhood, appropriate treatment should be administered. Walters sees the paediatrician as the person best qualified to determine the baby's potential and plan appropriate treatment in consultation with the parents. Since this approach does not deny the basic right to life, it has something to offer those who cannot accept the totally secular 'personhood' argument.

Neonatal nurses and midwives may feel that the approaches described above shed little light on decision-making in difficult situations. It is for each person to examine their own beliefs and standpoint and reach a position that they feel is justifiable and from which they can argue on behalf of the baby and family.

The extremely low birth weight baby

Case study

Jan C. was admitted to the labour ward in advanced labour at 23 weeks' gestation. This was her fourth pregnancy, the others having ended in miscarriages before 20 weeks. At 43 years of age she felt time was running out for her to achieve a successful outcome and was desperate for this baby to survive. She was seen by the consultant obstetrician·who told the couple that, if the baby were to deliver now, its chances of survival were so poor that the regional neonatal unit would not consider collecting it. The hospital's own special care unit would not be able to offer more than basic care to the baby. In spite of the couple's pleas for everything possible to be done, when the baby was born, weighing 500 g, he was wrapped in a blanket and given to his parents to cuddle until he died about half an hour later.

Treatment of low birth weight babies

The question of what treatment should be offered to babies born alive at gestations below twenty-five weeks or with birth weights of less than about 600 g is one of the ethical issues that confronts midwives and nurses working in delivery suites and neonatal intensive care units. Only in the last two decades has it been possible to contemplate the survival of babies born at such extremes of size or gestation. There are documented cases of very tiny babies surviving at home wrapped in cotton-wool and nursed beside the fire (Vaux, 1986) but these were the exception rather than the rule. In the majority of cases nature took its course, the baby died and the parents did not expect otherwise. Now technology exists to keep alive those who would otherwise die and the media fascination with these 'miracle babies' means that the public expects that every live-born baby should be given all available help.

However, survival rates for babies weighing between 500 and 750 g are only of the order of 30% and for gestations between 24 and 26 weeks about 50%. The incidence of significant handicap in survivors below 1000 g is about 15% in good intensive care units (Levene and Tudehope, 1993). Thus a very tiny, immature baby may be subjected to a great deal of pain and stress with only a small chance of surviving undamaged. Whereas, the need continually to improve techniques and treatments that 'push back the frontiers of science' and to be the first to save the smallest or youngest is prevalent (Battle, 1987).

Unfortunately, the decision over whether to resuscitate a small baby often falls to the junior doctor who is called to the delivery. It is helpful if clear guidelines exist about when resuscitation should not be attempted, because once started it can be difficult to halt the momentum (Paris and Kodish, 1993).

Ideally the decision about how the baby is to be treated should have been made before the delivery. If a senior paediatrician is informed when any woman is admitted in very preterm labour, her notes may be studied and the situation and probable outcome for the baby discussed with the family. Where there is doubt as to gestation the fetus should be fully monitored so that he or she is delivered in optimum condition (Avery, 1987) and the parents should be warned that resuscitation may not be appropriate. Avery suggests that the obviously immature fetus of 23 weeks' gestation or less, with fused eyes is probably a candidate for non-resuscitation but also concedes that, 'many would advocate not resuscitating babies of less than 600 g' (Avery, 1987). This is the approach followed in Scandinavian countries, where babies below a certain birth weight are not treated (Southwell and Archer-Duste, 1993). If such a small baby is delivered, the child may be given to its parents to cuddle until dying peacefully in their arms.

For the midwife or junior doctor faced with the unexpected arrival of a very small baby it is best if every effort is made to maintain the baby in good condition until a decision is made not to continue with resuscitation. A cold, acidotic, premature baby is at great risk of intraventricular haemorrhage, a major contributor to future disability, but if kept warm and oxygenated from the start a decision can always be made later not to proceed (Avery, 1987).

Withdrawing intensive care

Case study

Baby Catherine was born at 26 weeks' gestation to an unsupported mother with six other girls ranging in age from two to 16 years old.

By the time Catherine was five days old it was evident from brain scans that she had significant areas of brain damage. She was being ventilated and had some abnormal movements. The doctors advised that treatment should be discontinued but Catherine's mother became very distressed at this suggestion, saying that she did not want her baby killed.

Reasons for withdrawal of intensive care

Neonatal intensive care includes treatments such as assisted ventilation, total parenteral nutrition and exchange transfusion. Babies undergoing intensive care are overwhelmingly of low birth weight, but may also be term neonates with birth asphyxia, congenital abnormalities, infections or other illnesses. Adult survivors of intensive care have testified to the unpleasantness of the experience (Dunn, 1982) and there is no reason to suppose it is any different for a baby. It must therefore be realized that there might be occasions when intensive care is doing more harm than good for a particular baby. If the eventual outcome for the baby is likely to be poor, discontinuing treatment should be seen as an option. This was the situation with baby Catherine, where the staff caring for her believed that prolonging her life was not in her best interests because of the probable degree of brain damage she had suffered.

Debate usually centres on what constitutes a poor outcome and the importance of future 'quality of life'. Bissenden (1986) asserts that the issue of the baby's future quality of life cannot be avoided: 'to suggest that a person who can achieve a physical and mental age of no more than 2, will remain totally dependent, and will be unable to communicate can have a good quality of life is wrong.' This attitude would meet with sympathy from most quarters and the problem lies in assessing confidently and accurately the infant's prognosis and conveying it to the parents.

For the preterm baby the greatest danger probably comes from intraventricular haemorrhage and periventricular leucomalacia, both of which are consequences of hypoxic episodes before or after birth. Intraventricular haemorrhage has an incidence of up to 50% in babies of 1500 g or less (Levene and Tudehope, 1993). Both these conditions can be diagnosed by ultrasound and experience over a number of years has enabled a fairly accurate picture of long-term outcomes to be built up based on the correlation of scan results with post-mortem findings and follow-up studies (Bissenden, 1986). When a baby's scan picture is read in conjunction with assessment of its clinical condition, it becomes possible to make a prediction about the degree of handicap that the baby is likely to suffer and then for a decision to be made as to whether continued intensive care is appropriate. However, it may not be clear what weight to attach to certain handicaps; for example, does Down's merit non-treatment? (See Chapter 9.)

The question then arises as to who should make the decision. Some North American units use an advisory committee and Weir (1984) lists some advantages of this approach, such as ensuring partiality, resolving conflicts between professionals and safeguarding the baby's best interests. Bissenden (1986) is wary of the committee approach but would involve the family doctor and perhaps a psychologist. All would agree that the parents have a part to play, but disagree about the extent to which the family should have the final say. Some paediatricians and ethicists believe that the parents are the appropriate decision-makers (Weir, 1984) and some parents may share this belief. Lee and Morgan (1989) quote the parents of a baby born at $24\frac{1}{2}$ weeks weighing 800 g:

> ... he was 'saved' by the respirator to die 5 long, painful and expensive months later of the respirator's side effects. ... As Andrew's parents, we had a heightened sense of his suffering. Also, we feared the prospect of having to care for the rest of our lives for a pathetically handicapped and retarded child. If this is considered less than noble, what then is the appropriate label for the willingness to apply the latest experimental technology to salvage such a high-risk child and then to hand him over to the life-long care of someone else? We believe there is a moral and ethical problem of the most fundamental sort involved in a system which allows complicated decisions of this nature to be made unilaterally by people who do not have to live with the consequences of their decisions.

The parents' concern was over their involvement in decisions both to initiate and discontinue treatment. An English parent of a premature baby who developed severe cerebral palsy shares these sentiments:

> If a crisis in treatment does occur, we feel there should be more onus on an informed decision by parents about the next steps. However difficult and traumatic it is to decide to stop treatment, nothing can compare with the anguish that dominates the lives of parents with a severely handicapped child (Doyle, 1992).

Many professionals would question whether the burden of decision-making should fall upon the parents, who may still be in shock after the birth of a preterm baby and may be unable to discern the baby's best interests (Bissenden, 1986). There is also the worry that a parent may feel lifelong responsibility and guilt for deciding that treatment should be discontinued (Whyte, 1989). Some parents would share this view; one mother, after being asked whether her daughter's ventilator should be switched off, wrote: 'The despair I felt at that moment was bottomless . . . because I felt the whole responsibility had been heaped on to me and I could not see how I could make that decision and go on living with myself' (Braithwaite, 1984).

So, on balance, decisions are probably (and usually in the UK) best made by an informal 'committee' of those involved in caring for the baby. This includes both professionals and parents, acting upon what they feel is in the best interests of the baby, taking into account present condition and the likely prognosis.

Should other factors be taken into account, such as the cost to the taxpayer of a severely handicapped child who requires special education and care and will make no contribution to society? Vaux (1986) calls this the 'ethics of necessity' and believes that economic considerations should never override the best interests of the child. However, the 'cost' of caring for a severely handicapped child is not measured in monetary terms alone. The parents' relationship is often put under intolerable strain, older siblings may be relatively neglected as their parents' time is taken up with the handicapped child and further pregnancies may be shelved through fear of history repeating itself or simply because there is no time or energy left to cope with a new baby. The point made by the parents of Andrew (above) is a valid one; should a decision be made to start a course of action from which one is not prepared to withdraw if the desired outcome is not achieved, bearing in mind that others will have to 'pick up the pieces'?

What should be the role of the neonatal nurse or midwife working in the neonatal unit or, indeed, caring for the mother? The UKCC Code of Professional Conduct (UKCC, 1992) states that nurses and midwives should 'act always in such a manner as to promote and safeguard the interests and wellbeing of patients.' For the neonatal nurse this means taking seriously her role as the baby's advocate, speaking on the child's behalf when decisions are being made and protecting its best interests. It is therefore important that the nurse knows her baby well. Primary nursing can be a help in this, giving the nurse the best opportunity to familiarize herself with the baby's normal behaviour and reactions and to understand the family situation. It is not necessarily a comfortable role, the nurse may find herself in conflict with the doctors if she feels they are causing unnecessary suffering or if she believes their decision to stop intensive care is too hasty. She may disagree with parents who withhold permission for certain treatments or, conversely, as with baby Catherine's mother, insist that they want everything possible done to keep their baby alive.

One vital role the nurse can fulfil is to ensure that the lines of communication are kept open between all parties so that feelings can be aired in an atmosphere of trust. The nurses caring for baby Catherine encouraged her mother to talk to her priest and, with her permission, involved him in discussions about Catherine's future. With time to think things through and repeated explanations, Catherine's mother eventually decided that her daughter had suffered enough. The ventilator was switched off and the family had a couple of hours together before Catherine died peacefully in her mother's arms.

The midwife caring for the mother can probably do most by listening and familiarizing herself with what is happening to the baby in the neonatal unit. She can help the mother clarify her own views and can assist her in expressing these to those caring for the baby.

When all the views have been aired, someone has to take the responsibility for making the final decision and this is usually the consultant. Midwives and nurses then have an obligation to translate this into practice (Whyte, 1989), ensuring that the baby continues to receive the highest standard of care and to help the family cope with the consequences of the decision.

Killing or letting die

Case study

Baby John was born at term by Caesarean section following a placental abruption. He was severely asphyxiated, required ventilation and did not make any spontaneous respiratory effort. At two hours of age he began fitting and large amounts of sedation were required to control this. After several days the sedation was allowed to wear off so that

John's neurological state could be assessed: the convulsions had stopped but John appeared to be comatosed. His parents were told that his outlook was very poor and that in view of this it would be better to switch off the ventilator and allow John to die peacefully. They agreed to this; John was baptized, taken off the ventilator and given to them to hold. Unexpectedly, John began to breathe on his own. After a couple of days it became apparent that he was not going to die, although he remained very floppy and unresponsive. When there was no improvement after several weeks it was decided to remove John's nasogastric tube and only offer feeds if he cried. As John's parents watched him become thinner and dehydrated they asked if he could be given something to put him and them out of their misery.

How to treat the dying baby

In many cases once the baby is taken off the ventilator death will ensue in a matter of hours or even minutes. This gives the parents valuable time to cuddle the baby, take photographs of the whole family together and gain memories which they can carry away with them to assist later in the grieving process. For the nurse it is an opportunity to retrieve some of the futility of the situation by helping the family through a grieving process which, if handled skilfully, can leave them stronger and closer. One American nurse summed up her feelings:

> If there is no progress and in fact the kid is getting worse, isn't it better to let him die with some semblance of dignity and then spend your time with the family, helping them to cope and get on with life? I try to help them find a meaning and a purpose in their child's life no matter how short or miserable it may have been.... Maybe even looking into the future, things they can do to remember this baby and changes they can make in future pregnancies to prevent the same situation from recurring (Raines, 1993).

However, where the baby is not tiny and immature but a larger baby with an abnormality or birth asphyxia, switching off the ventilator may not be enough to ensure that death swiftly follows. What principles should govern the caring of these babies when survival is not desired but will continue if normal nursing care is given? This is perhaps one of the hardest situations to deal with in neonatal intensive care and is a cause of considerable stress to all those involved.

Whilst the withdrawal of mechanical life support may be seen as acceptable 'letting die', few would condone active measures to end the baby's life. However, this can leave a feeling that the worst of all outcomes has happened, namely, a slow and distressing death. In the end it has to be decided whether the baby is to be fed or not for, as Callahan (1986) put it, 'denial of nutrition may in the long run become the only effective way to make certain that . . . biologically tenacious patients actually die.' In a review of medical literature on the subject Rothenberg (1986) found that warmth, hygiene, food and fluids were normally considered to be part of basic care, while artificially supplied fluids or nutrition, via an intravenous infusion or nasogastric tube for example, were seen by some as life-support and in a similar category as ventilation. In the case of a preterm baby or a term baby with brain damage where there is no sucking reflex, not to give feeds via a nasogastric tube may be the equivalent to starving that child to death. Many nurses find this completely morally unacceptable (Lowes, 1993) and it rarely leads to an easy and dignified death as in the case of baby John. Each nurse and midwife needs to study the issues involved and decide upon her own position so that she can face the situation (Rothenberg, 1986). Doctors may ask for feeds to be withheld and, legally, nurses can follow this instruction without compromising their professional position (Lowes, 1993), but they have to look after the baby day by day and deal with the parents' anguish as they watch their child become dehydrated and wasted.

This is a situation which is best discussed openly and attempts should be made to formulate a care plan for the baby which truly meets all the child's needs and is acceptable to the majority of the carers. Whyte (1989) hopes that, 'with a team approach to care, nurses will be free to contribute to decision-making without fear of victimisation if they appear to be swimming against the tide.'

The question of analgesia and sedation also causes concern in relation to the baby who is dying. Unlike an adult a baby cannot say when experiencing pain or distress and it therefore becomes the responsibility of the carers to decide when treatment is required. Nurses who readily administer pain relief to babies post-surgery may be reluctant to do so if this may shorten the baby's life and there is little evidence of pain. Again, this situation needs to be aired openly and an acceptable course of action arrived at.

The baby with abnormalities

Case study

Baby Shane was born at 34 weeks with Down's syndrome. He was the first baby of a couple in their 20s. He was also found to have oesophageal atresia and a severe cardiac defect. The paediatric surgeon advised that his post-operative prognosis would be poor, even if he survived surgery, and was reluctant to operate. The neonatologist agreed and Shane was given 'TLC' on the neonatal unit by his parents and the staff until he died at 10 days old.

How to treat the baby with abnormalities

With the increased use of antenatal screening tests and ultrasound in pregnancy fewer babies with serious abnormalities are being delivered. Conditions that can be detected in early pregnancy and for which termination may be offered include spina bifida, hydrocephalus, polycystic kidneys, Down's syndrome and other chromosomal abnormalities. The birth of a baby with one of these abnormalities, undetected during the antenatal period, may come as even more of a shock to both parents and staff than one anticipated by a positive scan result. In some cases the defect is incompatible with survival beyond a few days and the parents can be given a firm prognosis and helped to cope with their infant's short life.

However in other cases, in fact with most of the conditions listed above, the baby may survive for years with or without surgical or other active treatment. A decision has to be made as to whether, and how much, treatment will promote a good quality of life. The selection for treatment of babies with handicapping conditions has probably been common practice for a good number of years. In England in the early 1970s Lorber, a paediatric surgeon in Sheffield, published a number of papers describing the results of the selective treatment of babies born with myelomeningocele (Weir, 1984). He based his decision to treat on a number of clinical criteria which would give an indication of the likely outcome for the baby if treatment was pursued.

Around the same time similar suggestions, that some handicapped babies should not be treated actively, were being published in the USA. Conditions mentioned in the North American papers included anencephaly, microcephaly, intestinal obstructions, severe birth asphyxia, Down's syndrome and spina bifida. The paediatricians involved tended to be influenced by the degree of neurological impairment resulting from the condition, and where this was considered to be substantial, treatment was usually withheld.

> In our view the most important medical criterion is the degree of abnormality, disease or damage to the central nervous system, especially the brain. If there is little or no prospect of brain function sufficient to allow a personal life of meaning and quality ... non-treatment seems the prudent course of action (Weir, 1984).

Other paediatricians on both sides of the Atlantic, writing in the 1970s, disagreed with these views. Zachary (1976), a colleague of Lorber's, believed that the majority of babies born with spina bifida should be given the care necessary to minimize their handicaps, including surgery: 'I believe that our patients, no matter how young or small they are, should receive the same consideration and expert help that would be considered normal in an adult.' It was pointed out by others that an untreated infant who survived, and no one was able to say that withholding treatment always led to the baby's death, might suffer more impairment than if he had been vigorously treated at the beginning (Weir, 1984).

Legal cases on either side of the Atlantic in the 1980s resulted in differing outcomes. In England in 1981 Dr Arthur was charged with murder after he prescribed sedation and the withholding of feeds for a baby with Down's syndrome whose parents had rejected him. Public opinion about the case was divided but Dr Arthur was acquitted by the jury, giving British paediatricians no legal guidance about the course of action to be taken in such cases. Selective non-treatment has become the accepted way of managing babies with abnormalities in most centres and aggressive efforts to prolong life by extensive surgery or other measures are rare. Some believe that this may lead to the withholding of treatment in too many cases, especially if advances in medical knowledge and techniques are not taken into account (Southwell and Archer-Duste, 1993).

In the USA in 1982 the parents of a baby with Down's syndrome, tracheo-oesophageal fistula and oesophageal atresia refused consent for surgery on the advice of their obstetrician. He then ordered the baby to be fed, knowing that this was likely to cause the baby's death from aspiration. When the nurses refused to carry out this instruction, lawyers acting for the baby sought a court order to authorize intravenous feeding. This was rejected and the baby (known as 'Baby Doe') subsequently died (Whyte, 1989).

The case provoked extensive public and medical debate and eventually resulted in the passing of legislation in 1985 to protect handicapped infants, the so-called 'Baby Doe' regulations. The 'withholding of medically indicated treatment from a disabled infant with a life-threatening condition' was prohibited unless it would merely prolong the act of dying and would not contribute to the infant's survival (Moreno, 1987).

While this law does not require that all handicapped babies should be treated, there is perhaps, as a result of this legislation, a greater tendency to overtreatment by paediatricians in the USA than by those in the UK. A British television programme shown in February 1995 (ITV, 3D, February 16th 1995) filmed a two-year-old anencephalic in the USA being kept alive with nasogastric feeds and resuscitation when she stopped breathing. This was at the insistence of her mother, backed up by court rulings. Whilst the mother's faith in the power of God eventually to heal her daughter was admirable, it is hard to imagine a similar situation occurring in the UK where, in the absence of specific legal guidelines, quality of life has become the overriding consideration and, in addition, parents do not usually have so much say about how much treatment is offered.

In the end, a combination of factors will probably determine what treatment is offered to a baby with a handicapping condition: the views of the neonatologist; the severity of the defect; the availability of surgical treatment; the views of the paediatric surgeon; the gestation of the infant and the parents' attitude. For instance, in the event of active treatment not being advised, a care plan should be devised that addresses all the baby's physical and emotional needs and those of the family. To ignore these needs is to convey the message that abnormality negates the value of the infant's life.

Ethical issues in the allocation of resources

Neonatal intensive care, in common with other critical care areas, is expensive. In 1984 Newns estimated the cost of a neonatal intensive care survivor of less than 1000 g to be £10 000; for babies who did not survive the cost was £1000 (Newns et al., 1984). However it can be argued that because of the potential lifespan of survivors, neonatal intensive care is relatively cheap. Where neonatal intensive care produces a child who will take its place in society, few would disagree that this is money well spent. It is when survivors require considerable help from the state in terms of special schooling or benefits that doubts are raised about the cost-effectiveness of neonatal units. As the NHS is increasingly expected to operate as a business, it can be anticipated that cost considerations will play a larger part in decisions about care.

The area of resources encompasses both staff and equipment and these are often in limited supply. Stories abound of parents who claim that their baby was taken off a ventilator to make room for another. Even if this is a rare occurrence when the baby concerned is undamaged, it is true that insufficient intensive care cots exist for all the neonates who require them and some form of 'rationing' does have to be used. This may simply be a refusal to consider for treatment any baby below a given weight or gestation. A 'first-come first-served' policy is also usual, which may mean that a larger, more mature baby (with a better chance of intact survival) cannot be accommodated because smaller and less mature babies are occupying the available cots and ventilators. It would usually be considered unethical to take one of these babies off the ventilator to make room for a baby with the better chance, but that baby is then denied any chance, at worst, or, at best, has to undergo the hazards of a longer journey to a unit with a space. The tendency is to try to squeeze the baby in, which can place unacceptable pressures on already stretched staff and jeopardize the care of all the other babies in the unit.

As the number of preterm multiple births increases as a result of fertility treatments (see Chapter 10), neonatal units could be faced with the problem of a set of triplets or quads taking over a number of ventilators, stretching resources to the limit and giving one family several babies while perhaps denying others even one. As much fertility treatment takes place away from NHS hospitals where the neonatal intensive care units are situated, little liaison between the two takes place and the arrival of a set of preterm multiples is to a neonatal unit what a major incident is to a casualty department, except that the preterm babies will take up beds for many weeks. The fact that these babies have been conceived with difficulty makes the desire to 'save' them stronger but places an immense strain on available resources.

Conclusion

Neonatal intensive care is a branch of nursing/midwifery that offers enormous rewards for those who work within it. To see a very immature baby leave for home with its parents after weeks of highly skilled care and to see the child return months later, smiling and apparently developing normally, makes all the hard work, tiredness and heat seem worthwhile. There is also the satisfaction of helping a family through bereavement and to know that everything possible has been done to help ease their pain and assist them to grieve fittingly.

What makes neonatal intensive care practitioners question their role is when they hear that a baby on whom they lavished care for weeks has developed a major handicap, or when they are asked to continue to ventilate a baby who has suffered severe brain damage but is being denied a peaceful, dignified death.

If those working in neonatal intensive care units, both nursing and medical staff, can foster an atmosphere of trust and open discussion, many of the ethical difficulties can be eased or avoided. Formal or informal support networks can provide opportunities to share the load, both for those who have to make difficult decisions and for those who have to carry them out. Each practitioner needs to develop her own philosophy based on wisdom and an understanding of the issues involved, so that she can provide the best service for the babies and families in her care.

References

Avery, G. (1987). Ethical dilemmas in the treatment of the extremely low birth weight infant. *Clin. Perinatol.*, **14** (2), 361–365.

Battle, C. (1987). Beyond the nursery door: the obligation to survivors of technology. *Clin. Perinatol.*, **14** (2), 417–427.

Bissenden, J. (1986). Ethical aspects of neonatal care. *Arch. Dis. Child.*, **61**, 639–641.

Braithwaite, S.(1984). The ethics of neonatology. *Nursing Times*, Jan. 25, 25–27.

Callahan, D. (1986). On feeding the dying. In, To feed or not to feed: that is the question and the ethical dilemma. *J. Paediatr. Nurs.*, **1** (4), 226–229.

Doyle, C. (1992). Dominic and the ethical tightrope. *The Daily Telegraph*, 1 September.

Dunn, A. (1982). The human factor. *Nursing Times*, **78** (12), 471–3.

Kuhse, H. and Singer, P. (1985). Handicapped babies: a right to life? *Nursing Mirror*, **160** (8), 17–20.

Lee, R. and Morgan, D. (eds) (1989). *Birthrights: law and ethics at the beginnings of life.* Routledge.

Levene, M. and Tudehope, D. (1993). *Essentials of Neonatal Medicine,* 2nd edition. Blackwell Scientific Publications.

Lowes, L. (1993). Ethical decision-making: theory to practice. *Paediatr. Nurs.,* 5 (9), 10–11.

Moreno, J. (1987). Ethical and legal issues in the care of the impaired newborn. *Clin. Perinatol.,* 14 (2), 345–360.

Newns, B., Drummond, M., Durbin, G. and Culley, P. (1984). Costs and outcomes in a regional neonatal intensive care unit. *Arch. Dis. Child.,* 59, 1064–1067.

Paris, J. and Kodish, E. (1993). Ethical issues. In *Neonatology for the Clinician* (J. Pomerance, and C. Richardson, eds), pp. 531–45. Appleton and Lange.

Raines, D. (1993). Deciding what to do when the patient can't speak. *Neonatal Network,* 12, 6, pp. 43–8.

Ramsey, P. (1982). Introduction. In *Infanticide and the Handicapped Newborn* D. Horan and M. Delahoyde, eds), pp. xv–xvii, Brigham Young University Press.

Rothenberg, L. S. (1986). To feed or not to feed: that is the question and the ethical dilemma. *J. Paediatr. Nurs.,* 1 (4), 226–229.

Southwell, S. and Archer-Duste, H. (1993). Ethical aspects of perinatal care. In *Comprehensive Neonatal Nursing* (C. Kenner, A. Brueggemeyer and L. Gunderson, eds), pp. 14–35. W. B. Saunders Company.

UKCC (1992). *Code of Professional Conduct for the Nurse, Midwife and Health Visitor.*

Vaux, K. L. (1986). Ethical issues in caring for tiny infants. *Clin. Perinatol.,* 13, 2, p. 477.

Walters, J. W. (1988). Approaches to ethical decision making in the neonatal intensive care unit. *Am. J. Dis. Child.,* 142, 825–830.

Weir, R. (1984). *Selective Non treatment of Handicapped Newborns.* Oxford University Press.

Whyte, D. A. (1989). Ethics in neonatal nursing. In *Ethics in Paediatric Nursing* (G. M. Brykcznska, ed.), pp. 23–41, Chapman and Hall.

Zachary, R. (1976). The neonatal surgeon. *Br. Med. J.,* 2, 869–70.

Chapter 8

Screening and the perfect baby

Janet Holt

Introduction

Screening and diagnostic tests to detect fetal abnormality are available to most women as part of prenatal care, and major advances in the field of prenatal diagnosis have been achieved in the last 15 years. The use of diagnostic tests is becoming more common; it is possible to detect more diseases and the tests themselves have become more accurate as old tests are refined and new ones developed. These advances have been made possible by improved medical technology but, as in so many other areas of health care where technology plays a vital role, ethical questions inevitably arise. The precise incidence of congenital abnormalities is difficult, if not impossible, to define. Many early spontaneous abortions are thought to be the result of abnormalities in the fetus, while other abnormalities may not be detected during pregnancy and may remain unrecognized until some time after birth. Congenital abnormalities are, however, relatively rare, with an estimated figure of about 2% of all fetuses having a major malformation (Chapple, 1994).

The aim of prenatal diagnosis is to detect congenital abnormalities and disease in the fetus. Such diseases and abnormalities can be divided into two large groups. Some are genetic diseases, such as Huntington's disease, thalassaemia or cystic fibrosis, and tests may be offered to women when there is a known family history. The other group of diseases includes neural tube defects and Down's syndrome, which are not genetic diseases, but certain women are known to be more at risk than others of having an affected fetus. Screening programmes have been developed at local and national levels to detect such diseases and abnormalities. If abnormalities are detected the diagnosis can be useful in three ways. First, the information allows parents to prepare both physically and psychologically for the birth of their baby. Second, it may be possible to instigate some form of treatment to correct the disease or abnormality either *in utero* or following delivery, and early diagnosis allows arrangements to be made. Finally, termination of the pregnancy may be considered. Although the practice of prenatal diagnosis encompasses all three purposes, Bewley (1994) states that: 'termination currently dominates management. In most societies, diseases of neonates and children are considered afflictions, and many tolerate abortion'.

Modern prenatal care allows screening for fetal abnormality using a variety of methods. An ultrasound scan is routinely offered to women around 18 weeks' gestation. A scan at this stage of pregnancy is useful because, as well as detecting structural abnormalities, the fetus can be measured to confirm the expected date of delivery, and multiple pregnancies and the location of the placenta can also be identified. The triple test, a blood test used to identify biochemical markers of Down's syndrome, is commonly offered to women at 16 weeks' gestation, but practices vary from hospital to hospital regarding which women are offered the test. The triple test gives women an individual predicted risk of having a baby with Down's syndrome, but cannot indicate if the fetus is definitely affected by Down's syndrome or not. Any woman considered to be high risk can then be offered amniocentesis where a sample of amniotic fluid is withdrawn, fetal cells within it cultured and examined, allowing an accurate diagnosis to be made. Some centres offer chorionic villus sampling (CVS), a technique that allows specimens of placental tissue to be taken and examined to identify chromosomal abnormalities. CVS is usually offered to woman where there is a family history of genetic disease or if the woman has previously given birth to an baby with congenital abnormalities. The risk of miscarriage is greater following CVS than amniocentesis and the procedure is costly in time and money so its use is usually restricted rather than being routinely available (Lilford *et al.*, 1991).

It could be argued that prenatal diagnosis, with its emphasis on detecting abnormal fetuses, lies more in the province of obstetrics rather than midwifery and is therefore not of concern to midwives. While this may be true, midwives caring for women in pregnancy may find themselves involved in the prenatal diagnostic process in different ways; for example, a midwife may provide information to the woman about the tests offered, she may be present while blood is taken, or an amniocentesis performed, or she may care for and deliver a woman undergoing a termination of pregnancy. It would therefore be difficult for a midwife not to encounter some aspect of prenatal diagnosis in her practice, either directly or indirectly. It is obvious that midwives need to be knowledgeable about the tests available and the procedures for carrying out these tests, but they should also be aware of the ethical questions raised by the practice of prenatal diagnosis.

Many ethical questions arise as a result of using prenatal diagnosis, the most obvious one surrounding the decision to terminate the pregnancy when an abnormal fetus is detected, but there are other problems to appraise; for example, we may want to ask what is an abnormality and how severe does it need to be to justify the pregnancy being terminated? What should we screen for: obvious diseases and abnormalities such as cystic fibrosis and neural tube defects, or less tangible conditions such as a genetic predisposition to developing cancer? Are we just simply seeking the 'perfect baby' and rejecting less than perfect fetuses, including those considered to be the wrong sex? What is the ethical justification for using screening programmes? Should health professionals be obliged to offer the tests to all women, or just those considered to be at risk? This chapter will attempt to address some of these questions by examining the justification for screening programmes and the moral and legal status of the fetus. What constitutes an abnormality, the implications for existing disabled people and the issues of eugenics will be explored, with particular reference to the slippery slope argument.

Prenatal screening programmes

It is not possible to offer a comprehensive service to every pregnant woman to test for all potential abnormalities as this would in practical terms be very difficult to achieve. Even if this were a reality, there is a danger that the fetus would be exposed to a greater risk of miscarriage as a result of the tests, than the chances of an abnormality being detected. Use of prenatal diagnosis therefore is restricted to those individuals in the population considered to be high risk; for example, the triple test may be offered to women followed by amniocentesis if the test shows a high risk that the fetus is affected by Down's syndrome, but the test is not necessarily offered to all pregnant women. Individual hospital trusts and health authorities have differing criteria and while some may offer the test to all women, others restrict its use particularly to those considered to be high risk but it is not clear how such practices can be justified morally.

The use of screening programmes to detect abnormalities can be justified by taking a consequentialist approach to what constitutes a right or wrong action. In this view, the action itself is not inherently right or wrong, but what is important is the consequence of performing the action. The consequentialist will act to try and produce the best consequences for all concerned; for example, suppose your aunt gives you a piece of jewellery that has been in your family for generations and is of great sentimental value. Some weeks later your house is burgled and all your jewellery is taken. Your aunt discovers that you have been burgled and asks if the piece of jewellery she gave you was stolen. You could be honest and tell her that unfortunately that particular piece of jewellery was taken; however, you know that she will be extremely upset about its loss. Alternatively, you could lie and tell her that this piece of jewellery was still in your possession; but is telling such a lie morally defensible? You may argue that by telling your aunt the truth, you will be honest, something which may be considered to be inherently good. However the consequence of your honest action would be to distress your aunt, which you could argue was wrong and should be avoided.

Overall you have to decide whether telling the truth is of greater importance than distressing your aunt, and the consequentialist would argue that lying to your aunt is morally defensible because by doing so you are acting to produce the most favourable consequence. This does not mean that consequentialists have no regard for honesty but that there are some situations when telling a lie can be the right action to take. In the same way, if the birth of healthy babies is preferred and the birth of babies with some form of disability is to be avoided, then to maximize preferences women at risk of having a disabled baby should be offered prenatal diagnostic tests. This may result in the abortion of an affected fetus which, it may be argued, is a bad action, but such an action can be justified if more favourable consequences are achieved. An example of a widely available screening programme is that which aims to detect fetuses with Down's syndrome.

The risks of having a child with Down's syndrome rises considerably when the woman is over 35 years old and women in this age group are routinely offered tests to detect Down's syndrome. However, the total number of births in women over the age of 35 is less than in the younger age group so that only 37% of babies with Down's syndrome are born to women over 35 and the percentages are even smaller in the maternal age group of 37–40 years (d'A Crawford, 1983). This means that the majority of babies with Down's syndrome are born to women under the age of 35. So even if it were possible to screen 100% of pregnant women over 35 years old and all affected fetuses were aborted, a considerable number of fetuses with Down's syndrome would go undetected. This is because such women would not be considered personally at risk and consequently may not be offered any diagnostic tests. Although this provides a useful service for the individual, it contradicts the broader consequentialist justification for screening programmes. If the birth of babies with Down's syndrome is to be avoided in society as a whole, then screening programmes need to be available to all women, not just those considered personally at risk.

The moral and legal status of the fetus

One of the most fundamental ethical problems in prenatal diagnosis is the link with the option of induced abortion. Opinions vary widely about the morality of abortion in general, ranging from the extreme conservative position which disapproves of abortion in any circumstances, to the extreme liberal position which approves of abortion in any circumstances. Between these two poles are a multitude of other opinions on the morality of abortion, particularly concerning pregnancy due to rape, the period of gestation when the abortion is to be carried out, the risk of pregnancy to the mother's health and fetal abnormality. Some argue, for example, that abortion should not be generally available, but may be used in certain specific circumstances such as in cases of fetal abnormality. This type of argument seems to suggest that abortion on these grounds differs to other types of abortion and is morally defensible.

The Abortion Act 1967 has recently been amended by section 37 of the Human Fertilization and Embryology Act 1990. Under this act, abortion is lawful if the pregnancy is less than 24 weeks advanced and the continuation of the pregnancy involves a risk of injury to the physical or mental health of the woman or of her existing children, greater than if the pregnancy were terminated. However the Act considers abortion on the grounds of fetal abnormality separately and allows abortion at any stage in the pregnancy when there is substantial risk that if the child were born it would suffer from such physical or mental abnormalities as to be seriously handicapped. What this means is that abortion in the vast majority of cases is only lawful when performed under 24 weeks of gestation, but in instances where fetal abnormality is detected abortion can be allowed at any stage in the pregnancy (Human Fertilization and Embryology Act 1990). This suggests that, in law at least, abortion performed on the grounds of fetal abnormality is viewed differently to other sorts of abortion.

In the same way that opinion may be split over the morality of abortion in general, there are also opposing views as to whether this abortion differs ethically from other types of abortion. These views can be considered from the position of the fetus, the parents and society in general. The opinion of the fetus may seem irrelevant as it cannot be said to be a self-conscious being, but as the fetus will develop into a child with some sort of disability it may be suggested that if the child is likely to experience a life of suffering, disadvantage or discrimination then it would be better not to be born at all. In the USA this position has been challenged in law, whereby disabled people have instigated legal proceedings against their parents for not aborting them when fetal abnormality was detected in pregnancy. The Court of Appeal ruled in *McKay* v. *Essex AHA* [1982] that such claims for wrongful life will not be allowed in England (Fletcher *et al.*, 1995).

One difficulty in trying to decide whether it is better to abort an abnormal fetus rather than allow a child to face a life of suffering is in determining how much suffering is too much, or which abnormalities and to what extent they are likely to disadvantage the child or adult in later life. It is easy to distinguish between the anencephalic fetus which will subsequently die following birth because there is no possible treatment, and the fetus with a cleft lip which can be successfully treated by surgery following delivery. Whereas little can be gained by the birth of an anencephalic fetus, the fetus with the cleft lip cannot be said to be facing a life of suffering or disadvantage. Far more complex are conditions such as Down's syndrome which affect individuals in many different ways. Some children with Down's syndrome have multiple abnormalities or profound learning disabilities and are unable to perform even the simplest tasks. Others receive mainstream education, become employed and form the usual social relationships. Using prenatal diagnosis, it is not possible to detect or predict what sort of effects Down's syndrome will have on the child or adult in later life.

In the majority of cases the results of prenatal diagnostic tests are not available in the early stages of pregnancy. For many women, the pregnancy has been planned or accepted and abortion is not an option under consideration. Following prenatal diagnosis, she (and her partner) will be faced with the decision whether to continue or terminate the pregnancy. Research seems to suggest that when the prognosis is poor, most women decide on termination of the pregnancy; for example in a study carried out by Drugan *et al.* (1990) 93% of women decided on termination when the fetus was discovered to have chromosomal abnormalities and a poor prognosis. The birth of a disabled child will have profound effects on a family, and the decision to continue with the pregnancy or not will have to be made taking such factors into consideration. The morality of abortion to the parents will depend upon their attitudes to abortion in general and their opinions on disability. For some individuals this may be a difficult, if not impossible, thing to do without experience and can still prove to be problematic even when parents have a disabled child. In a study of 78 parents of Down's syndrome children, there was disagreement among the parents about what constituted a severe handicap. For one woman in this study, having had a child classed as handicapped had altered her idea of what being handicapped really was (Shepherdson, 1983).

Ultimately parents may make a decision to terminate a pregnancy based on a reluctance to give birth to a child who will potentially face a life of suffering or discrimination. But is this reality the case? Do disabled children, adults and their carers experience miserable lives? If fetuses with abnormalities are aborted, is there an underlying assumption that they are less valuable than 'normal' fetuses and if so what are the implications of this for existing disabled people in society?

Implications for disabled people in society

Not all disabled children and adults have a congenital abnormality, but a proportion of this section of society as a whole are affected because of genetic disease or due to abnormal embryonic or fetal development. Some will be affected because of an abnormality that might have been detectable in pregnancy and selective abortion carried out. There may be many reasons why these people have been born with abnormalities rather than aborted. It may be that screening tests were not available to their mothers, that their mothers were not considered to be high risk or that abortion was rejected as an option. If selective abortion carried out for certain abnormalities in pregnancy can be justified, then we may want to ask if this will alter the attitude of society towards the disabled? Could it be that disabled people whose birth could have been prevented by the use of prenatal diagnosis and selective abortion may be considered less valuable and not given access to social and medical facilities?

Provisions for disabled people within society are positively encouraged. New buildings are designed for use by those using wheelchairs, old buildings are adapted as necessary, theatres and television use sign language and subtitles for the deaf. Many job advertisements carry a statement encouraging applications from disabled people, and recently in the UK there have been attempts to pass legislation protecting the rights of disabled people. Instead of shutting people with learning disabilities away from the rest of society in institutions, there has been a change of attitude towards caring for them in the community. It is perhaps obvious that people with special needs should have these needs catered for to minimize restrictions on their lifestyle imposed by their disability. This, however, seems to be inconsistent with the way that disabilities are viewed when selective abortion is considered. If an abortion is carried out to prevent the birth of a child who faces life disadvantaged in some way, then what is suggested is that it is better for that child not to be born rather than to be born with a disability. But the reasons that provisions are made for people with special needs is to improve the life of disabled people and if this can be done, then it does not make sense to suggest that such a life is not worth living at all. It may be argued that an increase in the use of selective abortion could mean that even less efforts would be made to provide for disabled people in society, as there would be fewer people to make provisions for. This, in turn, could alter the way that society views disabled people. Conversely, if there are fewer disabled people in society, then more could be done for them as there would be fewer people competing for the same resources. How realistic a proposition this is in the current economic climate is uncertain.

Irrespective of what tests and abortion facilities are offered to women in the future, it is unlikely that all congenital abnormalities will be eradicated either because, for some reason, the diagnosis was not made in pregnancy, or because some women refuse the option of selective abortion. It seems inconceivable that women, particularly in a European democratic society, would be forced by law to have prenatal diagnostic tests and selective abortion if necessary. This issue was recognized by the Court of Appeal in *McKay* v. *Essex AHA* [1982], which claimed that imposing a duty to abort would infringe principles of sanctity of life and devalue disabled members of society in general (Fletcher *et al.*, 1995).

At present selective abortion is tolerated at the same time as measures are encouraged to improve the status of disabled people within society. One reason for this may be that there has not been a sharp decline in the number of babies born with congenital abnormalities, but rather this has been a more gradual process causing less of an impact upon society. Regardless of this, researchers in the field of prenatal diagnosis aim to devise less invasive, less expensive tests that can be made available to more women, which in turn will doubtless further reduce the number of babies born with disabilities. The emphasis from the medical profession is placed on detection and abortion of abnormal fetuses. One study found that 41% of a sample of 210 consultant obstetricians agreed with the statement that: 'the state should not be expected to pay for the specialised care of a child with a severe handicap in cases where the parents had declined the offer of prenatal diagnosis of the handicap' (Farrant, 1985).

Although there does not appear at present to be any overt discrimination against disabled people or against women who knowingly give birth to a disabled baby, we cannot be certain that this will be the case in the future. Economic constraints and increased financial demands on an already overburdened health care system may lead to reduced care in the future.

Eugenics

Objections have been raised to prenatal diagnosis and selective abortion because it is a poorly disguised form of eugenics. Opponents of screening view it in this light as a 'seek-and-destroy mission' (Green *et al.*, 1992). In the late 19th century Francis Galton introduced the term eugenics from the Greek root meaning good in birth or noble in heredity. Galton intended to identify a science which improved human stock by giving: 'The more suitable races or strains of blood a better chance of prevailing speedily over the less suitable' (Galton cited in Kelves, 1985).

However noble Galton's original intentions might have been, eugenics became a controversial subject. It became associated with racist philosophies and the identification of individuals likely to indulge in criminal behaviour based on intelligence levels. The UK and the USA established eugenics societies and sterilization of people considered to be defective was permitted in some European countries and American states. The abuse of eugenics reached its peak during the Holocaust when millions of people with genetic profiles considered undesirable were murdered. Eugenics as a science subsequently became discredited, although some may argue that some forms of eugenic practices still continue.

Although there are two types of eugenic theories, positive and negative, only the latter are of interest in human genetics. Negative eugenics attempts to identify inferior genes in a population and eliminate them to reduce the incidence of inferior characteristics. It may be argued that prenatal diagnosis is a form of negative eugenics as defective genes are identified and attempts are made to reduce the incidence of genetically inherited diseases and abnormalities. If these practices are a form of eugenics, then it may be plausible that they should be as morally suspect as previous practices. However, this is dependent upon an assumption that eugenic theories always have sinister applications, which is not necessarily the case; for example, soon after birth all babies are tested for phenylketonuria (PKU), an inherited disease, which if left untreated causes severe learning disabilities. The test is relatively non-invasive, simple and inexpensive, but, of more importance, the disease can be successfully treated by dietary restriction. This form of screening programme can be considered to be negative eugenics, as by identifying a disease caused by a defective gene, inferior characteristics, in this case learning disabilities, can be avoided. Clearly, even the strictest opponents of eugenic theories would not object to this practice. The crucial issue here is that this practice benefits the child enormously by showing that although a defective gene is present, relatively simple treatment can be instigated to prevent profound disabilities. Similarly, some people are aware of the fact that they have a family history of a genetic disease, such as Huntington's disease, Tay–Sachs disease or cystic fibrosis. Prior to the woman becoming pregnant the couple may attend for genetic counselling where the risks of the fetus being affected can be assessed. If there is a high risk, some couples may decide not to have a child. This practice can also be described as negative eugenics, but again it is beneficial to the individuals concerned without harming others.

The historical connotations of eugenics in the quest to purify the gene pool make it a highly emotive subject, but if the sole aim of providing screening programmes to detect diseases like PKU is to improve the gene pool of the UK, then there seems little point in restricting the practice to diseases that can be treated, especially if such individuals would be able to produce children with the same genetic defect. The gene pool could be improved more effectively if such children were still treated, but then sterilized to prevent them reproducing in the future. It would be even more effective to screen for as many inherited diseases as possible even if treatments were not available and take measures to ensure that such people cannot reproduce. Clearly the aim in testing babies for PKU or providing genetic counselling for couples with a family history of genetic disease is not an attempt to purify the gene pool but to offer services of great benefit to individuals and is not morally questionable. When such practices do become morally questionable is when they are abused, legally enforced or lead to other less desirable practices.

Selective abortion is described as an abuse of eugenics because abortion on such grounds is seen as analogous to the genocide practised by the administration of the Third Reich. Although it may be argued that there are similarities between the two, it is not obvious that this is an appropriate analogy. The practice of genocide perpetrated by the Nazis was directed at improving the gene pool of the Aryan race on a national scale and people were forced to comply with the regulations. In the 1990s, undergoing prenatal diagnosis and selective abortion is a decision that individuals make for personal reasons without force and not to comply with any regulations.

Although a form of negative eugenics, it is possible to apply eugenic theories in ways that benefit society without any sinister undertones. Nevertheless, there still remains the possibility that these practices may be abused by forcing people to abort an abnormal fetus or by society adopting negative attitudes to disabled people. It may be argued that although prenatal diagnosis is not in itself morally questionable, by allowing the practice, we may progress down a slippery slope that will culminate in abusive practices in the future.

The slippery slope

This argument is frequently used by opponents of prenatal diagnosis and alleges that if one practice is allowed, then there will be a natural progression to other practices. Williams (1985) has described two different forms of the slippery slope argument, the 'horrible result argument' and the 'arbitrary result argument'. The 'horrible result' argument concerns what is at the bottom of the slope. Although the practice of prenatal diagnosis itself can be morally justified, there is a danger of a natural progression towards practices which are not; for example, detection of an anencephalic fetus may be morally permissible, but allowing selective abortion of the anencephalic fetus may subsequently lead to the detection and abortion of a fetus for a less acceptable reason, such as being the wrong gender, having the wrong physical characteristics or IQ. Supporters of this argument would suggest that the only way to ensure that society does not slide down the slippery slope towards this horrible result is not to allow prenatal diagnosis or selective abortion in the first place.

This argument may be significant because there have been clear cases of abuse in the past. We know that it is possible for abusive practices to occur and the memories of these past events are all too apparent. However, it may be argued that precisely because such abuses are remembered, then this memory in itself may serve to make people aware of the potential dangers and thereby prevent the repetition of such practices. It is, of course, impossible to disinvent practices. Although it may be decided that there is a strong case for the prevention of prenatal diagnosis because of what this practice may lead to, the knowledge of prenatal diagnostic techniques will remain along with the potential for abuse. Banning prenatal diagnosis and selective abortion may even be counterproductive, as failing to regulate practices for which the techniques are known may lead to their covert use.

The 'arbitrary result argument' suggests that once on the slippery slope any further discriminations will be arbitrary. If it is not morally acceptable to detect and abort a fetus because it is abnormal, then there are no further discriminations to be made. Alternatively, if this practice is considered to be morally acceptable, then it becomes necessary to decide what constitutes an abnormality. As stated previously, fetal abnormalities range from being incompatible with life to what can be described as minor physical defects with a wide range of variations in between. If an abnormality incompatible with life is detected, then there may seem little point in continuing with the pregnancy and so a distinction could be made between these cases and others. There are other situations when the outcome cannot be so clearly defined as, for example, in cases of spina bifida. Sometimes the abnormality is severe and the baby will die soon after birth, but in other cases the child may only be slightly affected or corrective surgery may be possible.

If prenatal diagnosis and selective abortion are allowed for some cases of fetal abnormality, then to draw the line between these and other abnormalities may seem to be arbitrary. In many areas of life we do resort to making arbitrary distinctions, such as the selection of 30 miles per hour as the speed limit for vehicles in residential areas. It may not be clear why this precise speed should be selected, but it is obvious that we should distinguish between safe and dangerous speeds for vehicles to travel at. In the same way it may be possible to distinguish between those abnormalities where detection and abortion would be permissible and those where it is not, for example between severe abnormalities and minor abnormalities. This would not help to solve the problem of difficult cases like spina bifida but it does not follow that because of difficult cases the practice should be abandoned altogether. Suppose that a traffic policeman observes one person driving at 31 miles per hour and another driving at 29 miles per hour. He may fine the first person but not the second, a harsh action when the distinction is so small. Like spina bifida this too is a difficult case, but it is unlikely that a suggestion of abolishing the speed regulations altogether would be considered a viable solution.

It is possible to detect the sex of embryos and fetuses and such information is useful in cases where abnormalities are sex-linked, such as Duchenne muscular dystrophy. Prenatal diagnosis in these cases may not be morally objectionable, but the information could also be used by parents to select the sex of their child on social rather than medical grounds. This is another formulation of the slippery slope argument involving:

- Practice A: prenatal diagnosis to determine the sex of the fetus for medical reasons;
- Practice B: prenatal diagnosis to determine the sex of the fetus for social reasons.

Practice A may not in itself be morally questionable, but it may lead to practice B, which is. There are several possible less desirable consequences of sex selection such as an imbalance of the sex ratio, increased conflict between the sexes, the setting of a precedent for genetic engineering to achieve eugenic goals and the potential for abuse by a totalitarian state (Motulsky and Murray, 1983). It has been suggested that sex selection has implications particularly for women, as male fetuses would be favoured above females but totally restricting the use of prenatal diagnosis and selective abortion would also have implications for women left to care for disabled children. It may be argued that the maintenance of reproductive freedom is of more importance than protecting women from the dangers of complete or partial femicide (Hayry, 1989).

Conclusion

There can be little doubt that the practice of prenatal diagnosis raises a multitude of ethical questions particularly pertaining to selective abortion of abnormal fetuses. Abortion on grounds of fetal abnormality is legally permissible and in law is considered separately from other types of abortion, however this does not make the practice morally acceptable. Prenatal screening programmes can be justified using a consequentialist approach to ethics, but inequalities in the availability of tests contradict this. Programmes can only be justified in this way if tests are available to all women without bias. For some, the search for the perfect baby is morally questionable, an application of negative eugenics theories, and may have implications for the way that disabled people are viewed in society. Undoubtedly conflict exists between current positive attitudes towards disabled people and aborting fetuses with the same disabilities. At present, we appear to be able to tolerate such conflicts, but against a backdrop of increasing demands on social and health care systems, can we be confident that such positive attitudes will continue? Or will the disabled and women who choose to give birth to disabled babies be discriminated against?

Perhaps prenatal diagnosis can be morally justified, but by allowing the practice, we will slide down the slippery slope towards less desirable practices. The fetus affected by Down's syndrome and aborted today may become the fetus of the wrong sex aborted tomorrow. It may be argued that the very fact that society is aware of the potential for abuse will serve to prevent this from becoming a reality, but whatever opinions are voiced, the knowledge, technology and techniques exist and there is a danger that restricting the use of prenatal diagnosis and subsequent selective abortion may lead to its covert use without proper regulation. This would be a serious form of abuse and clearly of little benefit to women or society as a whole.

References

Bewley, S. (1994). Ethical issues in prenatal diagnosis. In *Prenatal Diagnosis* (L. Abramsky and J. Chapple, eds), pp. 1–22, Chapman and Hall.

Chapple, J. (1994). Screening issues—the public health aspect. In *Prenatal Diagnosis* (L. Abramsky and J. Chapple, eds), pp. 54–69, Chapman and Hall.

d'A Crawford, M. (1983). Ethical and legal aspects of prenatal diagnosis. *Br. Med. Bull.*, **39**, pp. 310–14.

Drugan, A., Greb, A., Johnson, M. P. *et al.* (1990). Determinants of parents' decisions to abort for chromosome abnormalities. *Prenatal Diagnosis*, **10**, 483–490.

Farrant, W. (1985). "Who's for amniocentesis?" The politics of prenatal screening. In *The Politics of Reproduction.* (H. Homans, ed.), pp. 96–177, Gower.

Fletcher, N., Holt, J. Brazier, M. and Harris, J. (1995). *Ethics, Law and Nursing.* MUP.

Green, J., Statham, H. and Snowdon, C. (1992). Screening for abnormalities: attitudes and experiences. In *Obstetrics in the 1990's: Current Controversies* (T. Chard and M. P. M. Richards, eds), pp. 65–89.

Hayry, M. (1989). Selecting our offspring—some objections and counter objections. *Ethical Problems in Reproductive Medicine*, **1**, 36–38.

Human Fertilization and Embryology Act (1990). HMSO.

Kelves, D. J. (1985). *The Name of Eugenics.* Penguin Books.

Lilford, R. H., Irving, H., Gupta, J. K., *et al.* (1991). Transabdominal chorionic villus biopsy versus amniocentesis for diagnosis of aneuploidy: safety is not enough. In *The Embryo; Normal and Abnormal Development and Growth* (M. Chapman, G. Grudzinskas and T. Chard, eds), pp. 91–100, Springer.

Motulsky, A. G. and Murray, J. (1983). Will prenatal diagnosis with selective abortion affect society's attitude toward the handicapped? *Research Ethics*, **128**, 277–291.

Shepherdson, B. (1983). Abortion and euthanasia of Down's syndrome children; the parent's view. *J. Med. Ethics*, **9**, 152–157.

Williams, B. (1985). Which slopes are slippery? In *Moral Dilemmas in Modern Medicine* (M. Lockwood, ed.), pp. 126–137, Oxford University Press.

Chapter 9

Ethics of fetal tissue transplants

David Lamb

Introduction

Debates over the legal and ethical regulation of organ transplants in the past 20 years have focused primarily on the adult and infant brain-dead donor. Yet the use of tissue from aborted fetuses raises a number of new legal and ethical issues. Does the fetus require special protection? Is a discarded fetus equivalent to other forms of 'medical waste'? What is the moral status of the aborted fetus and whose consent should be sought for the use of fetal material? Do existing statutes and codes of practice adequately regulate the retrieval of aborted fetal tissue? There are questions concerning the link between induced abortions and the use of fetal tissue derived from them. Can the potential benefits of fetal tissue transplantation be insulated from the moral taint of abortion? To what extent can the dead, aborted fetus be regarded as morally equivalent to the brain-dead organ donor? Or is the fetus to be regarded as a donatable organ comparable to a kidney or liver? It cannot be both a donor and a donation. If, as some argue, it is morally equivalent to a person, then it could be said to be a donor, albeit an 'involuntary' one. If it is a donation, then its moral status is that of an organ. In many recent debates on the ethics of fetal tissue transplantation it is not always clear whether the fetus is given the moral status of a person or an organ. These issues are of relevance to midwives as they may be involved in caring for a woman undergoing a termination and be required to help explain the choices the woman might have to make. Further, debates concerning the status of the fetus are of central importance for midwives, as the attitude one adopts towards the fetus affects practice at every level.

Guidelines for the use of fetal material

The majority of commissions and investigative panels in recent years have concluded that the use of fetal tissue is ethical, provided that certain safeguards are in place. There have been 19 reports from commissions or investigative panels worldwide on the use of fetal tissue and experimentation. Although different in minor respects (for example, there are different recommendations concerning the father's consent to the use of fetal tissue and different procedures for obtaining consent for the use of material after elected and spontaneous abortions), most of them have recommended that fetal tissue should be honoured with the respect accorded to dead bodies (Coutts, 1993).

In the UK the Polkinghorne Committee, which reported in July 1989, outlined a Code of Practice which followed Sweden and the Netherlands in stressing the need for maternal consent. The committee also advocated a 'separation principle', namely that there must be 'a separation of the supply of fetal tissue from its use.' Thus there must be no direct contact between abortion clinics and fetal tissue researchers. This is designed to ensure that the need for fetal tissue does not influence the decision to have an abortion. The Polkinghorne Committee (1989) took the view that:

> whatever one's ethical opinion about abortion itself, it does not follow that morally there is an absolute prohibition on the ethical use of fetuses or fetal tissue from lawful abortion ... the termination of pregnancy and the subsequent use of fetal tissue should be recognised as separate moral questions and we regard it as of great importance that the separation of these moral issues should be reflected in the procedures employed ... great care should be taken to separate the decisions relating to abortion and the subsequent use of fetal material. The prior decision to carry out an abortion should be reached without consideration of the benefits of subsequent use.

According to the separation principle, informed maternal consent for tissue use must be sharply separated from the decision to terminate the pregnancy. The committee also recommended that the father's consent should not be required for the use of fetal material. The Polkinghorne Code of Practice was accepted by the Minister for Health and circulated to Health Authorities. It recommends that proposals to use fetal tissue for research and therapy must satisfy an ethics committee of the value of the research, indicate the absence of alternatives to the proposed use, and provide a demonstration that the researchers have the necessary facilities and skills to undertake the project.

Potential benefits of fetal tissue transplantation

In 1972 the Peel Report listed 53 ways in which research on fetal material could be of benefit. Since then there have been many more proposals that could be added to the list. The most immediate practical application of fetal tissue research is the transplantation of human fetal dopamine-secreting neurones to the brains of patients with Alzheimer's disease and medically unresponsive Parkinson's disease. The advantages of fetal material over other human tissue for transplantation purposes lie in its proliferative capacity and weak antigenicity. New applications are constantly sought. Recent use involves umbilical cells from fetuses as an alternative to bone-marrow transplantation, and research on fetal tissue could lead to therapies for infertility treatment and the prevention of many miscarriages. A more recent and controversial proposal involves the use of fetal ovarian tissue in fertility treatment. Although this procedure is not technically possible, and some medical researchers are sceptical about its future efficacy, strong public objections have been made. A report from the Human Fertilization and Embryology Authority (1994) referred to objections which included the perceived linkage with abortion, identity problems for children conceived in this manner, and fears that it would introduce steps towards the production of 'designer' babies. The report did, however, sanction the use of fetal ovarian tissue for research, provided that prior written consent was obtained from the woman undergoing an abortion after she had received adequate counselling.

Use of fetal tissue procured from legal and voluntarily undertaken abortions is justified with reference to the public good. Those who advocate the use of fetal tissue stress: that abortions would not be performed in order to meet a need for human tissue; that the abortions would take place whether or not fetal remains were useful; that it is better put to use for public benefit than destroyed; and that material from whole or living fetuses is not requested, only aggregates of cells from dead fetuses (BMA, 1988).

What, then, are the objections? Despite the potential benefits of fetal tissue transplantation a considerable number of ethical objections have been made, several of which will be examined below. The basic moral issue is not that new: it is whether certain human individuals can be exploited to obtain potential benefits for others. There is an increasing awareness that the dead fetus should be treated with respect and piety, and that it is not equivalent to 'medical waste'. In the UK religious services are performed for dead fetuses and the Health Council of the Netherlands (1994) noted that nowadays it is common for the parents' desire for the cremation of a fetus to be recognized and respected. The need for respect towards fetal remains is uncontested, as evident in guidelines developed for dealing with the product of late abortion. Philosophers who disregard the moral status of the fetus, with abstruse appeals to criteria for personal identity, have not even begun to recognize the moral issues involved. The most powerful objection to the use of fetal tissue is bound up with the ongoing controversy over the rights and wrongs of voluntary abortion. The source of the controversy lies in the fact that the tissue involved is derived from induced abortion, the morality of which continues to generate religious and moral disagreement.

Abortion and the separation principle

Can discussions about the potential benefits of fetal tissue research and transplantation be morally insulated from arguments about the rights and wrongs of induced abortions? Or is it necessary to have reached the conclusion that voluntary abortion is ethically acceptable before one can advance arguments in favour of fetal tissue transplantation? These questions have so far dominated the debate on both sides of the Atlantic.

Objections to fetal transplants include the arguments that it promotes a degrading attitude to human beings, and killing and dissecting a fetus is a violation of the rights of the developing human being and that participation in fetal transplantation will contribute to the brutalization of medical personnel. The Polkinghorne Committee (1989) denied this charge and argued that material derived from induced abortion carries no moral taint. This argument is not accepted by many pro-lifers who endorse the use of material if and only if it is taken from spontaneous abortions. This, however, would reduce the potential supply considerably, as material from spontaneous abortions is unsatisfactory because it carries a high risk of chromosomal abnormalities and a risk of viral infections. It is also an unsatisfactory source because of damage to the tissue due to the lapse of time between the death of the fetus and its expulsion from the uterus.

Neither side in the debate believes that the need for human tissue provides a justification for terminating a pregnancy. The point at issue is whether the rights and wrongs of abortion (usually portrayed in terms of competing interests between maternal choice and rights attributed to the developing human being) should be distinguished from arguments concerning the use and potential benefits of fetal tissue research and transplantation.

John Robertson (1988) employs an analogy with organs harvested from homicide victims in order to separate the benefits of fetal transplants from the moral taint of abortion. Pro-lifers certainly view abortion as equivalent to homicide. Yet no one suggests that the benefits derived from the procurement and distribution of organs from murder victims are morally tainted by the mode of death. Moreover, it would be absurd to suggest that surgeons and medical students who undertake research on legally obtained cadavers of murder victims are brutalized by their activities. According to this argument it would seem to be acceptable to benefit from what is perceived as an evil act without actually applauding the evil.

Another objection is that the potential benefits of fetal transplants may put pressure on women to conceive and abort in order to produce fetal tissue. One case, frequently cited in this context, involves the daughter of a man suffering from Alzheimer's disease who petitioned the courts in order to be inseminated with her father's sperm so as to provide him with fetal tissue for a neural transplant. This, however, is an isolated case and in many respects was an unnecessary request as neural tissue transplants lack antigenicity, thus obviating the need for a close genetic match between donor and recipient.

However, the case that fetal tissue transplantation will encourage induced abortion is strongly advanced and anti-abortionists argue that if the benefits are widely accepted then the public might become more favourably disposed towards abortion and less likely to support future legislation aimed at reducing the number of induced abortions. It is also argued that a woman in an ambivalent state about an abortion might just be tipped in favour by the utilitarian argument that benefit might accrue from it. Of course, these arguments depend on the respondent sharing the view that further curbs on abortion are morally supportable. Those campaigning for even greater relaxation of abortion laws would hardly endorse this standpoint.

Proponents of fetal tissue research and transplantation maintain that predictions of increased numbers of abortions are speculative and that among the many reasons why women choose abortion the desire to produce fetal tissue for therapeutic purposes is likely to remain insignificant. Yet if we grant a separation between arguments about the rights and wrongs of abortion and the beneficial uses of fetal tissue, supporters of greater relaxation of abortion laws could not appeal to the beneficial use of aborted fetal material as a moral justification for the abortion in the first place. On the other hand, for the anti-abortionist there *is* moral complicity: not active collaboration in the evil deed, maybe not even indirect association which suggests some form of approval, but the kind of moral complicity bound up with a failure to take steps in preventing that evil. This kind of complicity could be seen to survive the institutional safeguards – for example, avoidance of any connection between the abortion clinic and the transplant surgeons – designed to maintain the separation principle.

A further consideration of the morality of excising organs from brain-dead homicide and accident victims may be relevant at this point in the investigation. It can certainly be argued that there is no evidence to suggest that the growing need for adult cadaver organs has triggered an increase in homicide rates or impeded proposals to reduce mortality rates by means of seat belt regulations or curbs on the use of firearms. It can also be argued that demand for fetal tissue is unlikely to lead to an increase in the number of induced abortions. And just as one can see a reduction in murders and fatal road accidents as morally desirable whilst still benefiting from organs harvested from the victims, it would seem that one can maintain a standpoint of either neutrality or moral condemnation of abortion whilst condoning the benefits derived from the use of fetal remains.

If there is little difference between excising organs from homicide victims and aborted fetuses, then it would seem one can take either side in the dispute over the morality of induced abortion and still endorse the benefits of fetal tissue research. It should be noted, however, that endorsement of the separation principle requires that the fetus is regarded as an independent being, akin to an organ donor, not as an unwanted organ. This conclusion has implications for the problem of consent to fetal experimentation. What tips the argument against the appeal to moral taint is that it is potentially too embracing. Any use of human tissue can be linked to some form of evil, as tissue can be put to benefit when taken from the victims of homicide, road accidents, suicide, or the bodies of the poor. Yet there are no moral arguments that can link transplant surgeons with murderers, dangerous motorists, and the outcomes of an uncaring and unequal society. Despite strong feelings about the wrongness of abortion there is a long-established tradition of deriving benefit out of wrong: studies of the effects of poverty-induced disease and studies of victims of war and earthquakes have provided benefit, providing that those benefiting are not perpetrators of the original tragedy. However, this does mean that each case has to establish absence of complicity. Thus if a clear separation is to be maintained between the arguments concerning the moral status of abortion and arguments concerning the appropriate use of fetal tissue it is important that it is recognized that the elimination of any connection between the two procedures is conducted on a case-by-case basis, not by appeal to a once-and-for-all distinction.

Among the threats to the separation principle are practices where interests in the procurement of fetal material are allowed to influence the timing and method of pregnancy termination. It has been objected that fetal tissue transplantation may involve unnecessary risks to pregnant women if it leads to a situation where the date of the termination is determined by the desire to obtain satisfactory tissue.

There is a short answer to this objection: any decision taken with regard to the date of termination, once termination has been authorized, should be taken with reference to the interests of the mother alone. Any other course would be counter to well-established principles of individual care and the moral rationale underpinning legally performed abortions, namely the overriding interests of the mother.

Attention has been drawn to occasions where there have been modifications in the procedure for termination due to the need for fetal tissue. In one experimental study conducted in Sweden, which involved transplantation of human fetal brain tissue to rats, the method of terminating pregnancy was altered so as to enhance survival of the tissue. Thus: 'To obtain less damaged fetal tissue, the routine vacuum aspiration was slightly modified. After dilation of the cervical canal, but prior to suction, fetal tissue was removed by forceps' (Olsen et al., 1987). This kind of practice could have heralded a dangerous step towards the shifting of moral concern too much in the direction of those who require fetal tissue. There are, however, laws in Sweden which nowadays prevent doctors from varying methods of abortion to suit the convenience of people who want to use fetal tissue.

The fetus and the dead donor rule

Current research proposals are strictly related to the removal of tissues from dead fetuses. It is generally regarded as immoral to extract material from fetuses maintained *ex utero*, or to remove tissues from fetuses *in utero* before they are dead. Most guidelines recommend that the fetus to be aborted should be given the same protection as a dying organ donor, stressing that parts should not be removed from, and experiments should not be performed upon a living fetus. But in the face of a strong appeal to the potential benefits that can be derived from experiments upon living fetuses serious inroads into the 'dead donor rule' could be made. Why, it may be argued, should we wait for the fetus to be dead before experimentation is allowed, as it is already doomed because of the impending abortion process? Why wait upon its death before permission is sought for its dissection? If abortion is to be allowed, then why not end its life by the removal of vital parts for experimental or transplantation purposes? No doubt there are many benefits to be derived from such a course, but it is not the prime purpose of the moral philosopher to advocate *any* course of action insofar as potential benefit can be predicted. An extension of this proposal could quite easily reach sentenced criminals awaiting execution and children and others suffering from fatal injuries. The potential damage that could therefore be inflicted upon the moral status of transplant surgery should be carefully weighed, not to mention widespread moral indignation against harmful experiments upon the living, before such actions are tolerated. It is, of course, clearly obvious that any steps to legitimize the removal of organs from the soon-to-be-aborted fetus would undermine the separation principle, upon which rests the argument that fetal tissue transplantations can be morally insulated from arguments about the moral taint of abortion.

The fetus as a commodity

The potential use of fetal material has given expression to fears of 'an entire new bio-industry which is on the verge of coming into being just to secure and process (utilizing sterile and freezing techniques) fetal tissue and organs in order to make them available for commercial use' (White, 1994, unpublished observations). These fears are understandable, but this problem is not confined to the harvesting of fetal tissue; it is also a concern with regard to adult organ donation and proposals for the further use of human tissue. In recent years a small number of philosophers have argued in favour of a market approach to the procurement of human tissue on the utilitarian premise that the profit incentive would increase the much needed supply. Opponents argue that it is degrading to treat human parts as commodities.

There is very strong resistance to the idea that fetal material should be treated as a marketable commodity. Resistance to the sale of fetal material is bound up with beliefs that the fetus, as a developing human being, is 'entitled to respect, according it a status broadly comparable to a living person' (Polkinghorne Report, 1989). As a human being it is not an object that can be bought or sold. Neither fetuses nor children, alive or dead, can be regarded as chattels.

In many respects a fetus is dissimilar to an organ, tumour or discarded tissue, and arguments about the potential sale of human fetuses are not strictly similar to arguments in the current controversy over the potential sale of organs. If the fetus were similar, there would not be such a controversy over induced abortion. There may be objections to the removal of kidneys for commercial transactions but there are no pressure groups in support of the rights of a functioning kidney. A fetus is, even if it is unwanted, distinguished by the fact that it possesses a potential to become a member of a human moral community, that it possesses a genetic identity, and when dead, though smaller than a human cadaver, it merits a degree of respect. For this reason the United States' National Organ Transplant Act of 1984 was amended in 1988 to ban 'sales of fetal organs and subparts thereof'. The Health Council of the Netherlands (1994) recommend a principle of non-commercialization, and in the UK the Polkinghorne Report (1989) went even further than the Peel Report (1972), in its rejection of the profit motive, arguing against 'inducements' such as administrative costs or discounts on fees charged to the woman having an abortion.

One of the problems that has occurred when formulating ethical guidelines for fetal tissue transplantation is that it is not always clear whether writers on this subject view the fetus as an organ, like a kidney or liver, or whether they view it as a (developing) human being. If it is an organ, it can be donated. Moreover, if a case were established in favour of organ sales then, so the argument goes, a fetus could be sold. One philosopher, Kathleen Nolan (1988), was so exasperated by writers who confused fetuses with organs that she wrote a paper entitled 'Genüg ist genüg: A fetus is not a kidney'. She concluded that use of fetal material should be restricted to abortions performed on ectopic pregnancies, where removal of the fetus is undertaken because its development outside of the uterus places the mother in a life-threatening situation. According to Nolan this restriction guarantees that the benefits of fetal tissue transplants are separated from 'moral stigma' attached to abortion.

The problem of consent

Several objections have been raised against the proposal that maternal consent to fetal transplantation should be sought. Should a woman who has chosen to abort retain rights regarding the disposal of her fetus? Philosophers and lawyers are divided on this issue. Some argue that there is no moral basis for seeking the mother's consent to the use of fetal tissue. Others have argued that a decision to terminate a pregnancy is also an effective withdrawal of interest in the disposal of the fetal remains. 'Has she not already abdicated responsibility for the fetus by opting for abortion?' asks John Harris (1985). The fact that the fetus grows inside the body does not provide a basis for the creation of property rights. Similarly, argues Harris, viruses, tumours and bacteria grow in bodies without endowing the host with property rights over them. This position seems to regard the aborted fetus as a form of 'medical waste', equivalent to a placenta following childbirth or bone following surgery, which can then be put to some beneficial use. But public opinion is changing with regard to the further use of human tissue and at least one influential inquiry has recommended that consent is sought for *all* uses of human tissue (Health Council of the Netherlands, 1994).

Some philosophers and theologians argue that maternal authority extends only to decisions to terminate the pregnancy. In some cases this can even be separated from a decision to kill the fetus. Mason and McCall Smith (1991) point out that: 'There is in fact, no certainty that all women seeking a termination of pregnancy also seek the destruction of their fetus—indeed, one may wonder whether or not the woman's right to control her pregnancy extends to a right to control the destiny of a "viable" fetus.'

It is important to separate two concepts of abortion: termination of the pregnancy and killing of the fetus. These are morally distinct, although in early abortions termination of pregnancy involves killing the fetus. Later in pregnancy, however, the fetus could, with medical assistance, survive removal from the uterus. Arguments that support abortion on the grounds that a woman has the right to terminate an unwanted pregnancy may be covered by arguments supporting the first concept but might not be extended to her wish for the fetus to be dead; for example, several arguments in favour of termination of unwanted pregnancy often refer to one's right not to have one's body employed as a life-support for another being without consent. This argument could not be extended to grant a wish for the other being to be dead. Yet many arguments for abortion do express a desire beyond termination of pregnancy, to the desire not to be a parent in the biological sense. Should the mother's wish for the death of the fetus be respected? The resolution of this problem may well have some bearing on the problem of maternal authority over the disposal of aborted fetal tissue.

If one argues that the mother should give consent to the use of her fetus for experimental or transplantation purposes, it is important to indicate why. Does she give consent because the fetus is hers to donate, because it is a part of her body like a kidney or a bone marrow donation? Yet fetal tissues and organs are unlike organs which can be given up from her body; they are the organs of another body which has grown within her body. It is from the body of another individual. This important distinction has been employed to limit maternal authority over the disposal of fetal material. Proposals to limit maternal authority have been made by the Protestant theologian, Paul Ramsey (1975) who argues that, 'When a parent resolves to destroy her unborn, she abdicates her right to make decisions on the fetuses' behalf'. In a similar vein James Burtchaell (1989) has argued that: 'The decision to abort is an act of such violent abandonment of the maternal trust that no further exercise of such responsibility is admissible.' According to Burtchaell there are limits to parental authority which are bounded by the moral duties of guardianship. Hence: 'When a parent resolves to destroy her unborn she has abdicated her office and duty as guardian of her offspring and therefore forfeits her tutelary powers' (Burtchaell, 1989). Burtchaell also refers to a letter from former US President Ronald Reagan (personal communication to Joseph R. Stanton, MD, of the Value of Life

Committee, 1989), which says: 'The use of any aborted child for these purposes raises the most profound ethical issues, especially because the person who would ordinarily authorize such use—the parent—deliberately renounces parenthood by choosing an abortion.' On the other hand, denial of maternal authority might be construed as a punitive sanction against the mother for electing to abort. Arguments over the problem of maternal consent reveal just how difficult it is to separate the moral arguments over induced abortion from the proposed benefits of fetal transplantation. For if an analogy is established between human and fetal cadavers then consent from someone who is morally authorized to give it is required.

John Robertson (1988) argues that the case for denying maternal control is not persuasive: 'As a product of her body and potential heir that she has for her own compelling reasons chosen to abort, she may care deeply about whether fetal remains are contributed to research or therapy to help others'. Thus, Robertson (1988) goes on, 'she cannot insist that fetal remains be used for transplant because no donor has the right to require that intended donees accept anatomical gifts, but she should retain the existing legal right to veto use of fetal remains for transplant research or therapy. Her consent to donation of fetal tissue should be routinely sought.'

Another way of approaching the problem of consent turns on our views concerning respectful treatment of cadavers. If bodily parts are to be removed from a cadaver then respect for the cadaver requires either prior permission from the deceased (usually in the form of a donor card) or authorization from a guardian (usually a spouse or parent). If it is maintained, as some opponents of induced abortion do, that fetuses are persons, then a problem occurs. The one who has made the decision to destroy the fetus is also the very same person who is likely to be asked to act as guardian of its remains. In this respect, the issue of maternal consent is the crucial link between arguments about abortion and proposals for fetal tissue research and transplantation. An analogy here might be with a man who has just murdered his wife being invited to act as executor of her estate. There are, however, limits to this analogy and it is not clear what moral force it possesses. As Ruth Chadwick (1994) points out: 'This may not be a fair analogy, however. Surely the point is that the mother is thought, in cases of lawful abortion, to have the right to consent to the death of the fetus. The murderer is never thought to have such a right. The positions of the mother and the murderer are therefore fundamentally dissimilar.'

The argument about consent can be taken further. If those responsible for the abortion are prohibited from decisions concerning the use of fetal material, then authority over the disposal of the fetus must be withheld from the doctor or any other medical personnel involved in the abortion, as they too are involved in the destruction of the fetus. In any case doctors and hospitals have no grounds for exercising proprietal rights over the bodies of their former patients. Does this mean that authority should rest with the father? This too raises problems, admittedly of a different kind, as in many abortion decisions the father is unavailable or has already agreed to the abortion. In that case should authority lie with the Government or its agents, the courts or coroners? Objections have been raised against this proposal; by legitimizing abortion in the first place, so it is argued, the Government forfeits any moral claim to guardianship of the fetus. The consequences of this argument are ambiguous, i.e. that no one has any moral basis for the authorization of the use of fetal tissue. This, however is unsatisfactory as it could mean that no one should be allowed to use fetal tissue or that in the absence of any authority free use can be made of fetal tissue.

Conclusion

What should tilt the balance in favour of maternal consent is an understanding of the context and background to the abortion. Abortion is very often a dramatic experience. The sensitive nature of the fetus, its moral status, even when dead, is inescapably linked to the painful nature, for the woman concerned, of the circumstances of the abortion. In this respect there is a strong case for requesting maternal consent. Add to this a recognizable recent development in moral values where it is deemed to be appropriate to seek consent for further use of human tissue that was formerly regarded as 'medical waste'; for example, the report from the Health Council of the Netherlands (1994) recommends that consent should be obtained for any proposed use of human tissue. In cases involving aborted fetal tissue the report recommends that tissue can be used unless the woman, having been previously informed that it may be used, makes an objection. In the case of spontaneous abortion the report recommends that her express consent is required. Whilst this proposal rightly regards maternal consent to be essential it nevertheless draws an implicit and unnecessary distinction between procedures for consent or objection in the case of a wanted pregnancy and abortion in an unwanted pregnancy. If the public benefits derived from the use of fetal tissue are to be separated from any moral stigma associated with voluntary abortion, the way forward is to require express consent for any proposed use of fetal tissue.

References

BMA (1988). Medical ethics: Transplantation of foetal material. *Br. Med. J.*, **296**, p. 1410.

Burtchaell, J. (1989). The use of aborted fetal tissue in research and therapy. In *The Giving and Taking of Life: Essays Ethical* (J. Burtchaell, ed.), pp. 155–187, University of Notre Dame Press.

Chadwick, R. F. (1994). Corpses, recycling and therapeutic purposes. In *Death Rites: Law and Ethics at the Edge of Life* (R. Lee and D. Morgan, eds), pp. 54–71, Routledge.

Coutts, M. C. (1993). Fetal tissue research: Scope note 21. *Kennedy Institute of Ethics Journal*, **3** (1), 81–101.

Harris, J. (1985). *The Value of Life*. Routledge.

Health Council of the Netherlands: Committee on Human Tissue for Special Purposes (1994). *Proper Use of Human Tissue*. Health Council of the Netherlands.

Human Fertilization and Embryology Authority (1994). *Donated Ovarian Tissue in Embryological Research and Assisted Conception*. Human Fertilization and Embryology Authority.

Mason, J. J. and McCall Smith, R. A. (1991). *Law and Medical Ethics*, 3rd edition. Butterworths.

Nolan, K. (1988). Genüg ist genüg: A fetus is not a kidney, *Hastings Center Report*, December, 18, 6, pp. 13–19.

Olsen, L., Stromberg, I., Bygdeman, M., *et al.* Human fetal tissues grafted to rodent hosts: structural and functional observations of brain, adrenal and heart tissues *in oculo*. *Exp. Brain Res.*, **67**, 163–178.

Department of Health and Social Security (1972). *The Use of Fetuses and Fetal Material for Research*. Report of the Advisory Group (Peel Report). HMSO.

Polkinghorne Committee (1989). *Review of the Guidance on the Research Use of Fetuses and Fetal Material: The Polkinghorne Report*, HMSO.

Ramsey, P. (1975). *The Ethics of Fetal Research*. Yale University Press.

Robertson, J. A. (1988). Rights, symbolism and public policy in fetal tissue transplants. *Hastings Center Report*, **18** (6), 5–12.

Chapter 10

Reproductive technologies and midwifery

Lucy Frith

Introduction

Reproductive technology is an area of rapid change and expansion. There are new procedures and techniques reported with an unnerving regularity and it may seem to the midwife that it is almost impossible to keep up to date. This chapter aims to introduce the most common assisted conception procedures, to outline the role of the law and the relevant legislation in this area and to consider the main ethical dilemmas that have arisen from these scientific developments. Finally, the chapter will focus on areas where reproductive technologies could directly affect midwifery practice. Clearly, when dealing with such a huge area the chapter cannot hope to be exhaustive, but the main points of the debates and controversies will be highlighted and the reader directed to further sources.

Assisted reproduction procedures

In vitro fertilization (IVF)

Many people are familiar with the basic notion that IVF involves fertilization outside the woman's body; the combination of procedures that make up an IVF treatment cycle is probably less well known. The treatment cycle begins with the stimulation of the ovarian cycle with superovulatory drugs. This is deemed preferable to the natural cycle for two reasons; first, ovulation can be timed precisely, enabling the egg retrieval procedure to be scheduled in advance; and second, it produces multifollicular development and a greater number of oocytes can be retrieved. This is desirable, 'because pregnancy rates are higher with the transfer of more than one pre-embryo' (Ethics Committee of the American Fertility Society, 1994). The degree of superovulation is monitored by oestrogen assays and/or ultrasound scanning (RCOG, 1992). The oocytes are then retrieved, most commonly, by the transvaginal, ultrasound-guided route. This can be performed under sedation and is more favourable than retrieval techniques that need to be performed under general anaesthetic. The sperm and oocytes are then co-incubated for approximately 12–18 hours so that fertilization can occur. After 24 hours the embryos should have cleaved twice, to the four-cell stage, and then they are placed in the uterus transcervically by the means of a fine catheter.

Other techniques

The other most common infertility treatment is gamete intrafallopian transfer (GIFT). Eggs are collected in the same way as for IVF and then sperm and a maximum of three eggs are transferred together into one or both of the woman's fallopian tubes, replicating the site of natural fertilization. This process does not involve the creation of an embryo outside the body and is only suitable for women whose fallopian tubes are healthy.

Finally, it is worth mentioning donor insemination (DI). This is a very simple procedure by which a woman is inseminated artificially with donor sperm either at the cervical opening or in the cervical canal. This simple procedure requires no medical involvement; it is something that one could do at home with the help of a turkey baster (a tool often mentioned in the literature, although there may be other more suitable vehicles!). I shall now turn to the question of regulation.

Regulation and legislation

Scientific developments in embryology and techniques such as embryo transfer culminated in the birth of the world's first test-tube baby as a result of IVF in Britain in 1978. It was recognized that such developments, that concerned the very creation of life itself, had to be debated publicly and the ethical and social dimensions of these techniques assumed increasing importance. The Committee of Inquiry into Human Fertilization and Embryology (The Warnock Committee) was set up in 1982. The Warnock Committee reported in 1984 and recommended statutory regulation of medically assisted reproduction.

In 1990 the Human Fertilization and Embryology Act (1990) was passed to regulate such areas as embryo transfer, embryo research, the storage of gametes and embryos, the use in treatment of donated gametes (eggs and sperm) and of embryos produced outside the body. It was recognized, however, that in such a rapidly changing area it would be impossible to legislate for all future possibilities and developments, and that any legislation might quickly become out of date and hence unworkable in practice. So the Act provided for the creation of a regulatory body, the Human Fertilization and Embryology Authority (HFEA), continually to revise the provision of services and formulate policy on new developments.

It is worth noting that statutory regulation of medical procedures is by no means uncontroversial, as Kennedy and Grubb (1994) note: 'in general, particular aspects of medical practice are rarely regulated by statute in England. The 1990 Act is a significant exception to this; perhaps reflecting the fine balance between assisting the infertile and the fears of what could flow from the technologies as they are developed.' The USA, for instance, does not have similar all-encompassing legislation, leaving certain questions up to the discretion of individual doctors (Ethics Committee of the American Fertility Society, 1994). Such a response to the problems of assisted conception, namely legislation, could be attacked on the grounds that it limits the clinical freedom of doctors and scientists. It could be argued that the regulatory body is too blunt an instrument to oversee research adequately. As this is an area of such rapid development, there could be delays in research progress while the issues are debated publicly. However, in this area I would argue that the interests of scientists should not be allowed to override those of society. Constant questioning is needed because an appraisal of each new development is imperative to ensure that scientists practise in an ethical way.

It is now necessary to examine the role of the HFEA in more detail. The general functions of the HFEA are to act, '[a]s a regulatory body, much of the Authority's work relates to the inspection and licensing of centres carrying out *in vitro* fertilisation (IVF), donor insemination (DI) treatment or embryo research. The members of the Authority ensure that human embryos are used responsibly and that infertile patients are not exploited at a vulnerable time' (HFEA, 1994a). Thus the HFEA licenses treatment services and, 'stipulate[s] and set[s] standards for fertility centres and embryo research centres and license[s] only those which meet our criteria' (HFEA, 1994a). The HFEA normally inspects each licensed centre every year, unless there is a specific reason not to. The HFEA maintains a code of practice that gives guidance on the proper conduct of activities carried out under a licence (Human Fertilization and Embryology Act, 1990, s 25) and it also, 'monitors new developments in treatment and considers their risks and benefits, the skills needed to carry them out and whether they are necessary or desirable' (HFEA, 1994a).

The HFEA provides the very important function of not only reviewing the scientific desirability of procedures, but also considering the ethical acceptability of all aspects of assisted conception, 'respond[ing] to public concern about the social and ethical implications of new techniques' (HFEA, 1995a). It has done this by producing public consultation documents on certain issues, to date sex-selection (HFEA, 1993a) and donated ovarian tissue (HFEA, 1994b) (see Chapter 9). Such documents set out the issue to be considered, producing an overview of the main arguments (as perceived by the HFEA) and invite public response. It is here that both individuals and professional bodies can make their opinions known. However, despite the seemingly democratic nature of this process, the Sex-selection Public Consultation Document only produced approximately 200 replies from 2000 documents sent out, while the Donated Ovarian Tissue Document produced 25 000 requests for copies and some 9000 replies. Clearly, the general public have yet to feel involved in these decisions and although the donated ovarian tissue document produced a greater response, it is still a relatively small proportion of the general public.

Who is the parent?

Finally in this section on regulation it is worth clarifying the status of the parent as in certain situations, for instance egg donation, it might not be initially clear either who is the legal parent or what procedures need to be taken to establish legal parenthood.

The father: the husband of the woman undergoing such treatment is treated as the father of the resulting child, unless, 'it is shown that he did not consent to the placing in her of the embryo or the sperm and eggs or to her insemination (as the case may be)' (Human Fertilization and Embryology Act, 1990 s 28(2)(b)). This provision also extends to a couple who are not married, but receive the treatment services, 'together'(s 28(3)). Thus, the donor is, except in very rare circumstances (see Kennedy and Grubb, 1994) protected from becoming the legal father of any child born of his sperm.

The mother: under the terms of the 1990 Act the mother of the resulting child is: 'The woman who is carrying or has carried a child as a result of the placing in her of an embryo or of sperm and eggs, and no other woman, is to be treated as the mother of the child' (1990, Act, s 27(1)). Thus, it is the gestational function that determines legal motherhood, not the genetic relationship (i.e. if the woman receives a donated egg it is she, not the egg donor, who is deemed to be the mother).

In addition to this provision, Section 30 of the Human Fertilization and Embryology Act 1990 (the last remaining major section to be given effect) provides for maternal transfer of parental responsibility (Parental Orders Regulations 1994). This brings into effect new legal instruments called parental orders and concerns the cases of surrogate mothers. If a child is born to a surrogate mother then parental orders will allow the transfer of legal parental responsibility to the commissioning couple from the surrogate parent without the need for full adoption procedures. These orders can only be granted when the child is genetically related to at least one of the commissioning couple and the surrogate parents have consented no earlier than six weeks after the birth. (For more detailed information, see Kennedy and Grubb, 1994).

Ethical dilemmas

In a chapter of this size it is impossible to do justice to the range of ethical dilemmas that have arisen from the development of artificial reproductive technologies (ART). Hence, I want to concentrate on the main dilemmas that have exercised the policy makers when formulating the 1990 Act and those policy problems that have emerged since the passage of the legislation. I shall first consider the main ethical concerns that preceded the 1990 Act.

Prior to the 1990 Act there was considerable ethical debate about the acceptability of ART themselves. The Warnock Report characterized these as, 'opposition based on the fundamental principles ... of IVF ... that this practice represents a deviation from normal intercourse and that the unitive and procreative aspects of sexual intercourse should not be separated' (Warnock, 1984). The Report determined that this view should not be allowed to dictate policy because it was a matter of individual conscience, 'there will be those who will not wish to receive this form of treatment nor participate in its practice, but we would not rely on those arguments for the formulation of public policy' (Warnock, 1984). Hence, the fundamental principles that lie behind ART have been publicly accepted and the debate over whether to have such ART, in any form, has been superseded and replaced with debates concerning the type of regulation and how best to ensure that progress in ART proceeds ethically and responsibly.

A further area that was extensively debated in the Warnock Report was the use, storage and research protocols concerning embryos. Embryo research was an integral part of the scientific development of IVF and, in enabling embryos to be created outside the body, it has opened up a whole area of debate over the moral status of the embryo (Dyson and Harris, 1990; Singer *et al.*, 1990). The question is how to regard embryos in a moral sense, that is, some decision needs to be made as to what kind of entity they are, so that embryos can be treated in a morally appropriate way.

At one end of the spectrum, there are those who would claim that as the embryo is a human *being* it should be accorded full moral status and therefore be treated as you or I. The embryo thus has a right to life and this must be respected. At the other end, there are those who would contend that only human *persons* should be the recipient of moral status. Since personhood means a self-conscious, thinking, feeling being, the embryo is not a person, it is simply a collection of cells and it therefore has no right to life. There has been extensive philosophical debate over these issues and, as illustrated by the abortion debate, very little consensus has been reached (see Hursthouse, 1987).

Consequently, the Warnock Report framed the question in terms of, 'how is it right to treat the human embryo' (Warnock, 1984) and concluded that, 'the embryo of the human species should be afforded some protection in law.' This, in effect, was taking the middle ground, not according the embryo rights on a par with an adult, but not equating the embryo with a morally insignificant clump of cells. The Human Fertilization and Embryology Act 1990 adopted this position and states, 'a licence cannot authorise—keeping or using an embryo after the appearance of the primitive streak ... the primitive streak is to be taken to have appeared in an embryo not later than the end of the period of 14 days beginning with the day when the gametes are mixed' (s 3(3) & (4)). This 14-day cut-off point has attracted much criticism on the grounds that it is an arbitrary point of demarcation. Warnock has responded to this stating that, 'the point was not however the exact number of days chosen, but the absolute necessity for there being a limit set on the use of embryos' (Warnock, 1985). Thus, this setting of precise research guidelines, enshrined in legislation, has set a precedent in monitoring that the HFEA has followed (see HFEA, 1994c).

The creation and use of embryos has given rise to moral difficulties for many people and was arguably one of the main reasons why it was thought necessary to regulate ART. Those ART that do not involve the creation of embryos outside the body such as GIFT are not licensed by HFEA (unless they use donor gametes), although there has been an HFEA survey of GIFT clinics (HFEA, 1995a). I shall now turn to consider those ethical dilemmas unresolved by policy.

Access to ART

Since the passage of the 1990 Act two public consultation documents have been produced by the HFEA (1993a, 1994b) and the HFEA has determined, on the basis of this consultation, the current policy for these areas. An area where policy has not been conclusively formulated is the question of who should have access to ART and there has been increasing public and professional concern over this issue. Should ART be given to single women, non-heterosexual couples or post-menopausal women? The concerns here are often expressed in the form, 'are such people fit to be good parents?' The HFEA Code of Practice does not lay down any precise guidelines as to who should or should not receive infertility treatment. However, the well-being of the future children is held to be the paramount consideration. One of the conditions of a treatment licence is that, 'a woman shall not be provided with treatment services unless account has been taken of the welfare of any child who may be born as a result of the treatment' (Human Fertilization and Embryology Act 1990, s 13(5)). Thus, access to infertility treatment is only denied on the grounds that the future welfare of the child appears to be in jeopardy. This clearly leaves the matter to the discretion of the individual centres and practitioners, but the HFEA recommends that centres should have clear, written procedures to follow when assessing the future welfare of the child (HFEA, 1995b).

For single women and lesbian couples the sections of the Code of Practice that bear on their situation are, that in considering the welfare of the prospective child, 'the need of that child for a father' (HFEA, 1993b) is taken into account. But it is also stated that, 'where the child will have no legal father . . . centres should consider particularly whether there is anyone else . . . willing and able to share responsibility for meeting those needs.' This is a relatively progressive provision. Many countries (e.g. France) restrict access to married or stable heterosexual couples.

Another focus of concern has been the issue of whether post-menopausal women should receive infertility treatment. There have been various cases drawn to the attention of the public by the media, most notably the clinic in Italy that treated a 62-year-old woman, believed to be the oldest such mother. In April 1995 a 51-year-old woman gave birth to a daughter after receiving a donor egg. She had lied about her age so that she would be accepted for treatment, telling the clinic she was 47. Should these women have received infertility treatment?

In answering this question, one possible place to start is to consider the welfare of the future child. Is it self-evidently harmful for a child to have parents who are older than the norm? This raises the problem of what we consider the normal age for child-bearing. The Family Policy Studies Centre (1995) stated, in a report examining the birth rate, that more women are delaying having children until their late 30s and early 40s. The normal age to have children appears to be slowly rising. Thus, it seems to be almost impossible to determine what is the normal age for child-bearing in a society where changing social circumstances and improvements in health can shift that point.

Clearly, in considering the acceptability of treatment for older women, it is a matter of degree. We might think that 60 is too old, but 50 is just acceptable. This creates the problem of how we are to justify these two different limits. In response to this, there have been attempts made to determine a suitable cut-off point after which treatment should not be given.

There could be two cases that present themselves to infertility clinics, those women who require egg donation (for IVF) and those women who can use their own eggs. The women who require egg donation may not be those in the 'older' bracket (this will be determined as over 50 (HFEA, 1994a)). They might have a high risk of transmitting a serious genetic disease or they may have undergone a premature menopause. However, if a woman is post-menopausal she will require egg donation in order to conceive. It is argued that this could be used as a cut-off point for those seeking ART. If the woman has reached the menopause, then her fertile time is over (biologically) and this would provide an objective, testable point that was not subject to the individual practitioner's interpretation and judgement.

However, this seemingly straightforward solution masks two difficult problems. First, some women, albeit a very few, menopause prematurely, sometimes in their 20s. Would we then want to say that a woman in this situation is not to receive treatment? The response to this might be that we mean the average age of menopause and not the menopause itself, but this throws the debate back to interpreting norms and deciding who should have treatment purely on the grounds of age. A woman of 40 years old who has reached menopause may think that is too early, so how are we to distinguish between her and the 20-year-old when deciding who should get treatment if not by age?

Second, it has been argued that, 'age related decline in fecundity is associated with the age of the oocytes rather than the age of the uterus' (Abdalla et al., 1993). Thus, women of, say, over 40, although they may have not yet reached menopause, may wish to have donor eggs provided to minimize the risk of miscarriage. Thus, menopause ceases to be an important cut off-point as with the use of donor eggs women can conceive after their menopause. Again, the problem comes back to making the judgement of whether to treat on the basis of an individual's age, rather than a biologically determined point.

There is also the issue of scarce resources; this is a practical consideration but allocation is frequently based on the debates that have just been discussed concerning who should mother. Even if we accept in principle that there is nothing inherently wrong with providing treatment for 'older women', due to the shortage of donor eggs many have argued that younger women should be given priority. The Lister Hospital, which treated the 51-year-old in 1995, said that they had 600 women waiting for matched eggs and their main concern was that reports of older women giving birth would put off prospective egg donors. Further, with limited resources provided for infertility treatment within the NHS (ISSUE, 1993), again decisions will have to be made on which individual is to be treated.

However, to say younger women should be given priority either in treatment or to receive eggs, is again to make the decision turn on the age of the woman. Either we accept that there is nothing inherently wrong with older mothers and therefore do not discriminate when allocating resources, or we accept that there is something problematic about older mothers and seek to provide guidelines as to what is a suitable age limit for treatment. A precise age limit is always going to be problematical, but age 50 years seems to be the working limit of many centres. The HFEA states, in relation to this problem: 'The Authority believes that each case should be considered individually, bearing in mind the welfare of the child and all the implications for the couple concerned' (HFEA, 1994a). It makes the point that there are very few women over 50 who have been treated, but says, '[there] would be concern if a centre were repeatedly treating older women and would require the centre to justify this practice in terms of the welfare of the child' (HFEA, 1994a). This implies that as long as it is a rare event, then there is no need to make guidelines, but this does not indicate general support for treatment for those over 50. Maybe the best way to proceed is to keep the HFEA policy of considering every case on its merits, such as perceived ability to care for the child for a reasonable number of years, health of the woman and her partner, existing children and reasons for wanting the pregnancy, rather than trying to determine some age limit for treatment. Any age limit will be an arbitrary one and difficult to justify.

This section has not covered all the ethical dilemmas created by ART. The development of such technologies has forced us to think about our rights to reproduce, who should reproduce and what constitutes parental relationships to name a few. These are all questions that are important independently of ART, but ART have posed them with an urgency that has not existed before. It is also worth noting that these discussions have implications for general considerations of parental suitability, and so on, and conclusions reached for ART situations can illuminate other areas of concern.

Midwifery and reproductive technologies

Midwives will not be the professionals actively involved in the process of ART. This might lead them to suppose that this subject has no relevance to their profession. However, there are two reasons why a consideration of ART is of use to the midwife. First, midwives, as members of a profession concerned with women and childbirth, should have a general interest in all related areas so that they can take part in public debate on the issues and be able to offer appropriate advice to women in their care. Second, births that result from ART have to be managed and it is here that the midwife could become involved. The number of births resulting from ART in the UK is still very small, 3089 in 1993 (HFEA, 1995a). It is likely that in the future this number will rise not only due to more women seeking treatment but it is possible that the success rates of ART will increase, thus producing more births. I will now outline some of the ethical concerns that could be raised by caring for women pregnant as a result of ART.

Confidentiality

The midwife is bound by the duty of maintaining confidentiality for all her patients, but for those patients who have received ART there are additional provisions set out in the 1990 Act and the Human Fertilization and Embryology (Disclosure of Information) Act 1992. The two main concerns of the 1990 Act were to make sure that the child born as a result of ART did not find out inadvertently that it was conceived in this way and to protect the anonymity of donors.

Those involved in the care of a woman who has conceived as a result of ART have no automatic right to be informed of the circumstances surrounding the conception. The woman is under no obligation to tell her carers. Information can be disclosed but only with the consent of the person to whom the information relates and this is subject to clear controls and safeguards. Before the treatment centre discloses any information, reasonable steps must be taken to explain the implications of the disclosure, consent must be obtained in writing and, 'it is the person's right to decide what information will be passed on and to whom' (HFEA,1993b). A woman has full control over the information the obstetric team receives. The only exception to this is in the case of an emergency, but if it is practicable to obtain consent for disclosure and this is refused then information must not be disclosed. Once the information has been disclosed it 'is no longer covered by the special provisions of the Act, but only by the ordinary law on confidentiality' (HFEA, 1993b).

These confidentiality provisions affect the midwife in two ways. First, as the information regarding infertility treatment is covered by a specific statute, any disclosure must be sanctioned by the person to whom the information relates. It is not accessible under the general provision that professionals involved in a patient's care can have access to that patient's information. Thus the information that the midwife might receive could be very limited and she would be unable to attain more even if she felt it was in the patient's best interests. To illustrate this point consider the following hypothetical situation. The midwife might have been told that this is an ART pregnancy by the woman, who has authorized the disclosure of information relating to the drug protocols used in the superovulatory treatment. The midwife becomes concerned about the woman's husband who seems depressed and unwilling to provide any support to his wife. The midwife wonders if the cause of his depression is that he is not the genetic father of the baby. The midwife would like to know if her assessment is correct so that she can recommend appropriate counselling for the couple. The woman is very distressed but refuses the midwife's overtures to talk about the situation. However, the midwife cannot find out if the woman has received donor sperm without asking the woman for authorization, which she is reluctant to do due to the woman's distress, even though she thinks it would be in the patient's best interest if she had this information. Thus, this confidentiality provision removes from the midwife a measure of clinical autonomy, as it is left up to the client to decide what information should be shared.

Second, as stated, once disclosure has taken place it is no longer covered by the Act. Hence the HFEA (1993b) advises that: 'Centres should as far as possible ensure that those receiving information record details of treatment services only on the client's medical record and not on that of any resulting child.' This is to prevent a child learning 'in an inappropriate way that he or she was born as a result of treatment service.' So even though the midwife is not under the jurisdiction of the Act, she should be aware of the spirit of the provisions and aim to protect the child from an inadvertent discovery.

The pregnancy

In the management of an ART pregnancy there is the possibility of certain problems arising (which I shall cover below) of which the midwife should be aware. This is not to say that all ART pregnancies will be problematic, but simply that there are some potential pitfalls and if the midwife is sensitive to the possibility then this could provide a better basis for care and support for the woman.

There has been considerable dispute over the contention that all ART pregnancies are necessarily high risk. The HFEA overall attitude (that is reflected in the confidentiality provisions) is that there is no reason why those managing the birth should be aware of the circumstances of the pregnancy. This assumes there are no particular risks associated with such conceptions. If there are any risks, it could be argued that these are secondary to the treatment, that is, older women and multiple births, and these will be apparent to the midwife. In contrast, it has been argued that: 'A history of infertility, and particularly a pregnancy resulting from assisted conception should be regarded as a high risk factor in pregnancy' (McFaul et al., 1993).

The purpose of this discussion is not to come to a firm conclusion as to which of these risk assessments is correct. That would be beyond the bounds of this chapter. The purpose is simply to highlight the *possible* risks that the woman may be subject to, recognizing that not all women will be determined high risk. The ethical implications of these risk assessments will be considered; for instance, if ART are deemed to produce very high-risk pregnancies with little hope of good outcomes this could tell against the ethical acceptability of ART. I shall consider the issues raised by each stage of pregnancy.

The overall success rate for such treatments is still relatively low and this could affect the attitude of the woman and her general well-being throughout the pregnancy. Clearly, any couple receiving ART will have had a history of infertility and will have been trying for some time to have a baby. Once accepted for ART there is still no guarantee that a pregnancy will be achieved. In 1993 out of 21 823 treatment cycles, there were 3921 clinical pregnancies and 3098 live births. Per treatment cycle there is an 18·0% clinical pregnancy rate and a 14·2% live birth rate (HFEA, 1995a). Thus, even if a pregnancy takes place there is still a likelihood of miscarriage. Most women undergo a number of treatment cycles (outlined earlier) before pregnancy is achieved and this contributes to the stress and strain on the couple. Because of this low success rate it has been argued that ART cannot be seen as a therapeutic procedure but rather as an area of research (Spallone, 1989; Rowland, 1993). This raises the ethical question, is it justified to offer ART to women on the grounds that they will receive a therapeutic procedure when they are more accurately taking part in a research project? In order to answer this question it is necessary to come to a decision about acceptable levels of success rates, i.e. when is a success rate so low that the technique is still at the research stage? It could also be argued that if ART are still at the research stage then the midwife is unknowingly involved in a research project. This could compromise her professional autonomy as she is not being given the choice as to whether she wishes to participate and the midwife may feel uneasy about aiding the involvement of her patients in a research enterprise dressed up as a therapeutic procedure.

Hence, factors such as low success rates and a history of infertility could all make the pregnancy resulting from ART a very anxious time for the mother. The cause of the infertility could also make the woman more vulnerable to miscarriage during the pregnancy (see Joels and Wardle, 1994a) and although all these elements may not be recorded on the patient's notes, they must be borne in mind. Thus, understanding and an awareness of such factors can help form the basis for the kind of support the woman needs. Support requirements will be different for every woman and by getting to know the woman and by the amount of information she chooses to disclose, individual requirements can be gauged.

There are also risks to the woman in undergoing ART, for instance the danger of ovarian hyperstimulation syndrome which 'is a major complication of ovulation induction. . . . The most severe forms can be life threatening' (Tiitinen *et al.*, 1995). There have also been speculative articles that suggest repeated superovulation could be associated with an increase in ovarian carcinoma and this 'is being kept under review' (RCOG, 1992). As ART have a relatively short history it is still too early to evaluate the full extent of the risks. These are concerns that will affect other health carers more directly than midwives, but still concerns of which midwives should be aware.

To turn now to the pregnancy itself, there are two factors that often put the ART pregnancy automatically into a high-risk category: first, the women are more likely to be elderly primigravidae; the average age for ART was 34 years of age (HFEA, 1994a); and second, they are more likely to have multiple pregnancies. The multiple birth rate was 31·4% for ART compared to 1·25% in the overall population (HFEA, 1994a). Both these factors increase the risk of complications throughout the pregnancy. These risks could be determined without any specific disclosure of how the pregnancy was achieved.

Bound up with the issues of the risk status of the pregnancy are the possible effects on the provision of neonatal intensive care. One study (McFaul et al., 1993) found that the incidence of preterm births was higher among those who had received ART:

> The high rate of spontaneous preterm labour is in part the result of a high incidence of multiple pregnancy. It may also reflect the effect of ovarian hyperstimulation which results in the uterine environment being exposed to supra-physiological levels of sex steroids at the time of implantation.

Thus a higher demand for neonatal care may be apparent in hospitals that provide ART and the planning of maternity services must take into account the demands such pregnancies might make.

The types of risks, that might not be apparent to the midwife without specific disclosure, could affect the clinical decision of where the birth should take place; for instance, if a midwife has no knowledge that the woman she is attending has had ART and this woman asks for a home birth the midwife could decide (on the limited information she has) that this is acceptable. But this decision is not made on the basis of all the facts and it could be said that asking a midwife to make a clinical decision in these circumstances is compromising her clinical autonomy. For here the midwife has agreed to a place of confinement that is inappropriate for a pregnancy of such risk status and has been prevented from exercising her clinical judgement adequately. Thus, it could be said that the likelihood of risk factors coupled with stringent confidentiality provisions can put midwives in a very difficult position.

As Page states (1995), an important goal of midwifery is to prepare the woman for parenthood and an ART pregnancy could present distinctive demands in this area that need to be ascertained in consultation with the mother. Once birth has taken place, the adjustment to motherhood may be harder to make after such a pregnancy. 'She is more likely than usual to require support and there is evidence that post-partum depression is more common in women whose pregnancies have resulted from assisted conception' (Joels and Wardle, 1994b). However, it has been argued that couples who conceive in this way are more prepared for parenthood, and one study argued that the quality of parenting in families with a child conceived by ART is superior to that of families who have naturally conceived children (Golombok *et al.*, 1993). The implications of this study are far from clear, but I think it would be fair to say that as all children conceived by ART are very much wanted, this bodes well for the quality of parenthood they will receive.

Finally, it is worth noting that frequently a child born as a result of ART may not be the genetic child of one or both of the parents. How this affects the bonds between children and parents is not yet well researched, but it is imperative to be aware of this situation and comments like 'she really looks like her dad' may be very hurtful when the genetic father is unknown to the couple if donor sperm has been used.

In summary, ART pregnancies are often very fraught and stressful events for the couple and the midwife needs to be sensitive to the distinctive needs of such a couple. By being aware of the wider issues and problems raised by ART she can provide appropriate and skilful care in these cases.

Conclusion

This chapter has attempted to give a broad overview of the kind of ethical issues raised by ART. It has also tried to illustrate the distinctive problems that managing these pregnancies might create for the midwife. It is crucial that midwives follow the debates over ART so that, as individuals and through their professional bodies, they can ensure that these technologies proceed in a way that is beneficial and not harmful to the women who receive them.

References

Abdalla, H. I., Burton, G., Kirland, A. and Johnson, M. R. (1993). Age, pregnancy and miscarriage: uterine versus ovarian factors. *Hum. Reprod.*, **8** (9), 1512–1517.

Dyson, A. and Harris, J. (1990). *Experiments on Embryos*. Routledge.

Ethics Committee of the American Fertility Society (1994). Ethical Considerations of ART. *Fertil. Steril.* **62** (5).

Family Policy Studies Centre. (1995). *Bulletin*.

Golombok, S., Lock, R., Bish, A. and Murray, C. (1993). The quality of parenting in families created by new reproductive technologies. *J. Psychosom. Obstet. Gynaecol.*, **14**, 17–22.

HFEA. (1993a). *Sex Selection: Public Consultation Document*.

HFEA. (1993b). *Code of Practice*.

HFEA. (1994a). *Third Annual Report*.

HFEA. (1994b). *Donated Ovarian Tissue in Embryo research & Assisted Conception Public Consultation Document*.

HFEA. (1994c). *Donated Ovarian Tissue in Embryo research & Assisted Conception Report*.

HFEA. (1995a). *Fourth Annual Report*.

HFEA. (1995b). *Revised Cose of Practice*.

Human Fertilization and Embryology Act. (1990). HMSO.

Human Fertilization and Embryology (Disclosure of Information) Act (1992). HMSO.

Hursthouse, R. (1987). *Beginning Lives*. Blackwell.

ISSUE. (1993). *Infertility: the real costs*. The National Fertility Association, Birmingham.

Joels, L. and Wardle, P. (1994a). Causes and treatment of infertility. *Br. J. Midwifery*, **2** (9), 423–429.

Joels, L. and Wardle, P. (1994b). Assisted conception and the midwife. *Br. J. Midwifery*, **2** (9), 429–435.

Kennedy, I. and Grubb, A. (1994). *Medical Law*. Text with materials. Butterworths.

McFaul, P. B., Patel, N. and Mills, J. (1993). An audit of obstetric outcome of 148 consecutive pregnancies from assisted conception: implications for neonatal services. *Br. J. Obstet. Gynaecol.*, **100**, 820–825.

Page, L. (1995). Putting principles into practice. In *Effective Group Practice in Midwifery* (L. Page, ed.), Blackwell Science.

RCOG. (1992). *Infertility: Guidelines for Practice*. RCOG Press.

Rowland, R. (1993). *Living Laboratories: Women and Reproductive Technologies*. Cedar.

Singer, P., Kuhse, H., Buckle, S., Dawson, K. and Kasima, P. (1990). *Embryo Experimentation*. Cambridge University Press.

Spallone, P. (1989). *Beyond Conception: The new politics of reproduction*. MacMillan Education.

Tiitinen, A., Husa, L., Tulppala, M. and Simberg, N. (1995). The effect of cryopreservation in prevention of ovarian hyperstimulation syndrome. *Br. J. Obstet. Gynaecol.*, **102**, 326–320.

Warnock, M. (1984). *Report of the Committee of Inquiry into Fertilization & Embryology*. Cmnd 9314.

Warnock, M. (1985). *A Question of Life*. Basil Blackwell.

Part Three

Professional Issues

11

Ethical decision-making and the positive use of codes

Jane Pritchard

Introduction

In this chapter I will look at the role of codes of practice in a professional context generally and then consider their particular use in midwifery. Prior to this, the historical and legal framework will be mentioned briefly in order to illustrate how codes can have an especially important role for midwives, many of whom practise independently. What constitutes a profession is not uncontentious and it will be necessary to give an indication of what I understand by that term. In that context and in order to justify the place of midwifery amongst the professions, what midwifery is will need to be addressed. The place of ethical theory will then be discussed in relation to professionalism, and how it can be applied to midwifery. It will be argued that codes of professional conduct are most effective when used in combination with effective training in ethical decision making.

It may be useful to note that codes of practice are not all homogeneous entities and can be divided into different categories. Harris (1989) states that codes can be said to fall into three categories. He points out that the three categories he identifies are not consistently used throughout professions but simply illustrate the type and function of the various documents. The three categories are *codes of ethics*, which contain very broad ethical principles, for example, midwives should be beneficent, but there would be no mention of how or what this means in practice; *codes of conduct*, which contain more specific guidelines for actual behaviour, for example, such a document is inward looking and is intended for members of a particular profession; and *codes of practice*, whereby the professional body (or, indeed, industry) warrants certain standards of care or service to its clients generally. Such a code of practice is not unlike a customer charter.

Midwifery as a profession

Midwifery, arguably, is the only predominantly female profession given legislative endorsement. Men 'allowed' women to practise as midwives without male supervision. Apparently worried by the danger of witchcraft, certain stipulations were made as to how practice should be conducted. These became the Midwives Rules, which still have statutory force, albeit in their modern form. By contrast, codes of conduct are not legally binding in themselves but would be supportive evidence of good practice in, for example, negligence proceedings in a court of law. Their most immediate disciplinary force is with internal hearings for alleged breaches of the code held by the UKCC. All UKCC documents are referred to as the 'code' unless the context requires otherwise, when the named document will be stated and these include Advertising (March 1985), Confidentiality (April 1987), Exercising Accountability (March 1989), Standards for Records and Record Keeping (April 1993), Midwives Rules (November 1993), The Midwife's Code of Practice (May 1994).

Unlike most other professionals, for example doctors and solicitors, a midwife's practice is closely monitored throughout her career. This is done by midwifery supervisors who visit midwives while at work. Midwives have long had to take compulsory updating courses, whilst for other professions, for example solicitors, continuing education is a recent innovation. In this way practice is not only safeguarded against irregularities but uniformity is ensured from area to area. The supervisor will often compare actual practice with the recommendations for practice set out in the midwives code. Thus in midwifery, at least, the code is an everyday working guide. As such it has tremendous potential, particularly for independent midwives who might otherwise feel isolated, and it can be used as a helpful 'companion'. The profession would do well to stress this image of the code rather than the less positive images, i.e. seeing the code as a watchdog, or viewing it as too theoretical and not applicable in practice. These more negative images are sometimes appropriate and in the main do not help midwives to cement their position as autonomous professionals who can operate with minimal involvement from obstetricians in the majority of cases.

The fact that individual midwives have always been closely monitored could be viewed as evidence against midwifery being a profession in its own right and seen rather as a branch of medicine. If this is true, it is true in the sense that both solicitors and barristers are branches of the law having their own clearly defined areas of responsibility, but are still seen as distinct professions. For instance, under the Courts and Legal Services Act 1990, some solicitors are being licensed to have a right of audience in the higher courts, whereas previously that right was the exclusive privilege of barristers. This does not of itself argue against the professional status of either branch of the law but rather seeks to let the rights follow the type of work actually undertaken. It acknowledges that there may be some overlap of responsibilities 'near the edges' of the professions. Similarly, there may be areas of overlap between obstetrics and midwifery, both being a branch of medicine. One of the difficulties faced by midwives in their insistence on professional status has been that these edges have been allowed to become blurred, partly due to the increased use of technology in childbirth, for example, the increased number of Caesarean births in recent years (Francome *et al.*, 1993). In summary, the fact that the area of responsibility of a particular profession, in this case midwifery, has limitations is not seen as precluding that speciality from professional status. Midwives specialize in 'normal' births just as obstetricians specialize in 'abnormal' births but in these separate domains both can be termed professionals.

In Airaksinen's (1994) analysis of a profession he states that there must be some essential good in the aim of that profession in order to constitute such a classification. In the case of medicine, health is the 'internal value'. Nobody would deny, he argues, that health is not only a desirable but also a necessary good. In order for midwifery to be constituted as a profession it must have some good value that is not detachable from its practice, in other words, it must have some intrinsic good. That something is intrinsically good is sometimes difficult to grasp. It is made more difficult in some ways by the modern emphasis on standards of practice. We get used to standards changing and so we think of practice as being about skills which can be learned from time to time which are 'detachable from practice' because they change. To say that a profession has an intrinsic good must mean that this good does not change. What this unchanging aspect is can be the intention to do good and the fulfilling of that goal. Thus, the means to achieve the good may change with scientific and medical advancement, but the ends, the final goal, remain the same. While all professions share an intention to do good for their clients, individual professions have specialities. It is in those specialities that the particular values of a profession lie. What is 'good' for a particular profession is assessed in terms of how well or badly those special values are promoted.

When discussing whether midwifery is a profession, it is necessary to ask whether it is essential to childbirth that midwives practise. Strictly, the answer is probably not; mothers will give birth regardless of the presence of a person qualified to assist them, but to use an analogy from Airaksinen (1994), without doctors '[w]e just suffer and die'. Similarly, without midwives, mothers just give birth. If we use this argument that what constitutes the nature of a profession is the providing of some 'good', it can be claimed that when a midwife is involved her skilled mediation is an undeniable good. The fact that there may nevertheless be disasters that occur notwithstanding her involvement does not undo the good role of her presence.

It has been argued that midwifery is a profession and the special value or good of this particular profession needs to be elucidated. The aim of this chapter is to show that 'good' in the context of midwifery is 'skilled mediation' in childbirth. This is the involvement of the midwife in facilitating client choice over the type of birth and care she receives. In order to fulfil this intrinsic good the midwife must also continue to use all her skill and judgement to decide what options are realistically available for any particular client. Midwives are presently limited in their practice to normal births, by which we mean that when irregularities occur the midwife must hand over conduct of the case to an obstetrician or other medical practitioner but for the majority of their cases the client is healthy and able to make certain choices. In this sense it is argued that client choice is an ethical option for midwifery and on that basis skilled mediation is an intrinsic good that helps women have a fulfilling experience of childbirth. Hence, midwifery is correctly called a profession.

Ethics and popular ethical theories

Codes of ethics and/or conduct give guidance on how a midwife can arrive at 'good' practice. Good is used to indicate how competence will be determined and also what will be understood as being moral in the context of the midwife's values in her practice. Before what is good can be determined there must be an understanding of the ethical theories that may underpin or are reflected in the codes of practice.

Probably the most common ethical theories to be discussed in the context of health care are Kantian deontology and utilitarianism. With an increased emphasis on care in the community communitarianism can be added to these. While it is not the primary function of this chapter to discuss the formal philosophical theories, by way of clarification, what the writer understands by these terms should be briefly identified. These theories can be seen as 'silk screens' which are placed over the facts. Thus it is likely that the same facts when looked at through the priorities of the different screens will realize a different action to produce a good solution. By using a screen of priorities advocated by, for example, utilitarianism, what is right and wrong will be assessed in terms of the degree to which the greatest happiness has been brought to the largest number of people. By contrast, the screen used by a Kantian deontologist will understand right in terms of the professional doing her duty for the patient to the best of her ability without regard to competing needs or indeed consequences. A communitarian screen would view, for example, issues like confidentiality as having important implications for the community as well as the individual client. If keeping a client's confidence, for instance, could jeopardize the safety or 'good' of another or the wider community the right action might be to breach the confidentiality of the client.

When we talk about the unique values of a particular profession, what we mean is that the professional body and/or the midwives should agree the values of the profession. Thus if mediation in the light of client choice is the central value to midwifery, then 'good' action is decided in terms of how much a particular circumstance promotes that value. Skilled mediation in regard to client choice can be seen as a moral 'screen' for midwifery. In other words, by identifying the criteria and values of the profession it should be possible to work out how to solve a moral dilemma and decide what is right for this profession.

An important aspect of training to be a professional is learning the values of that profession and thus learning what is good in the terms of that profession's practice. The health service has long been familiar with the four principles. Let us imagine these acting like sub-screens, once more coming between the facts and the midwife who is trying to decide what it is ethical to do.

Prioritizing the principles

While most people will quite readily be persuaded that the principles of autonomy, justice, beneficence, non-maleficence and equal opportunity (not always added), and there may be others, are worthy ideals, a great deal of difference can emerge by ascribing a different priority to each. If beneficence is held to be most important, for example, the resulting action will be very different from an ethical position which holds justice to be most important. Professionals have, by definition (Koehn, 1994), an inclination towards the good, that is, to do what is ethical, but each profession must decide what priority or value it puts upon each principle. Promoting health is held central to medicine (Thomson, 1953) which arguably puts beneficence first. For midwifery, it will be argued that autonomy is the central principle, the principle that most closely aligns to mediation in regard to client choice.

The arrangement of the principles will depend on what theoretical approach to ethics is adopted. Ethics is understood as the study of determining what moral position is appropriate. It may be decided, for example, that there is a universal morality that can provide moral answers to all people on all occasions or, alternatively, it may be decided that this is too large a task and it is more appropriate to try to determine what is moral in a particular setting. If the former model is sought, it might be assumed that everybody, including people starting training for midwifery, will have some sense of morality. In this scenario ethical training for midwives would not be different from training for anybody else. In a multicultural society like the UK today, it is suggested that this cannot realistically be assumed. It is not within the remit of this chapter to define universal morality and it is not assumed that midwives share values automatically. In any event, training in ethics is as much about learning to think in a particular analytical way as about identifying what may or may not be moral in any given circumstance. On the latter model midwives must determine what is moral for midwifery. They themselves must identify what values are appropriate for their profession. Once agreed, there will be a framework in which to solve moral dilemmas in midwifery practice. In order for codes of ethics and conduct to be workable they should be consistent with the ethics of midwifery.

However, codes are not always made in such a conscious or consistent way; there is a tendency for codes to respond to cases in practice that have gone wrong. Advice is thus provided so that similar situations can be avoided in future. Thus codes have tended to be reactive rather than proactive documents. This is perhaps a necessary evil but is possibly why inconsistencies can occur. It is very difficult to make general rules from particular cases, as actual circumstances will never be repeated. This possibility highlights the need for codes to be used together with training in ethics. In this way, the thinking processes behind the rules will become more accessible as well as knowledge of the guidelines themselves. Thus the midwife will be well prepared to adapt rules to apply to different circumstances.

If codes develop in this way, it is likely that they will reflect several different ethical positions rather than be based consistently on one. This is not necessarily a bad thing but it is another factor that can make knowing what to do in practice unclear. This is likely to be especially true for the UKCC which has to accommodate the needs of three different professions.

Harris (1994) holds that the most common ethical position to be reflected in professional codes is a Kantian one. This is consistent with the characteristic of professionals (Koehn, 1994) that the intention behind an act is more important than the outcome. An emphasis on outcome rather than motive would of course tip the scales towards a consequentialist or utilitarian standpoint. Harris (1994) points out an inconsistency with Kantian theory in that the moral imperatives are imposed upon the midwife by the external professional body rather than being individually worked out by the rational agent (the midwife); but as Chadwick (1994) says, this can be the focus for improvement rather than a reason for dismissing the Kantian framework. One way in which such improvement could be realized is by incorporating into ethical training a full discussion of the values set out in the code. In this way, although the values are not individually conceived, they can be accepted and ratified by each midwife in practice.

This feature of codes, that they are motive centric rather than consequentialist, is significant and arguably goes a long way towards explaining the tension between professionals and management. It can be said that management as a tool of business (Pritchard, in press) is more likely to be governed by an end-oriented philosophy than by a concentration on motive. Management may well consider this preoccupation with intention time consuming and even sentimental.

Thus the tension between professionalism and management is real. One of the most common problems facing midwives in practice, particularly those attached to hospitals, is that guidance received from the professional body, possibly via the code or associated circulars, is inconsistent with the requirements of management expressed, for example in a hospital protocol. It is an example of a philosophical dilemma; the respective parties may have always to agree to differ.

There will be other moral tensions in práctice, because different bodies have their own intrinsic values, different professionals acting morally within their own values inevitably will disagree. This tension is at the heart of moral dilemmas. I have implied that doctors and nurses are likely to have different priorities from midwives and also the client. When talking about client choice this tension between professional and client may well centre upon issues of autonomy. The next section does not necessarily show an orthodox view of autonomy but seeks to find practical ways to find moral answers.

Making sense of autonomy

Clearly if a policy of client choice is going to be made central to the ethics of midwifery then the principle of autonomy must be thoroughly understood. Autonomy is the practitioner's right to make her own decisions in relation to her clients without interference from doctors. It is also used in relation to the client/mother's right to choose procedures and/or treatments which she feels are best for her. If such rivalling autonomies are not to lead to deadlock, the meaning of autonomy must be expanded beyond self interest.

It will be argued here that autonomy is negotiated choice, that the accountability tag so often hung on autonomy indicates the need to find a balance between having one's opinions overridden and having one's choices implemented. The exercising of autonomy sensibly must follow Aristotle's doctrine of the mean, that virtue is neither too much nor too little (Hutchinson, 1995). Thus autonomy in terms of client choice is not a client choosing whimsically from a menu of treatment options, some of which might jeopardize the midwife's own autonomy, but rather it is agreeing a course of action that will allow both client and professional to feel comfortable and both trust that the 'right' treatment has been carried out. The now infamous case (see Chapter 2) where a client refused to get out of the bath before delivery which resulted in the two midwives attending being suspended is a clear example of client autonomy being irresponsibly exercised to the detriment of that of the midwives. It is also an example of only one principle being applied to the exclusion of others. Autonomy may be the most important principle to midwifery but it must be exercised in the light of justice, beneficence, and so on.

Practitioners must act

One of the most difficult tasks facing the professional is that theory must always be translated into action. That ethical theories can lead to different answers is at the heart of the frustration between learning philosophical approaches and actually making decisions in practice. It is not uncommon for an experienced practitioner when asked why she adopted a certain course of action to say that she acted instinctively. While this may seem to be what happened (even to the midwife herself) it is altogether more likely that the decision was made, albeit quickly, in the light of well-learned practice and a deeply internalized belief in what constitutes right action. Arguably this is what Hunt (1994) means when he criticizes philosophers for 'teaching morality' to health professionals. Unfortunately, along with the seeming 'gut reaction' comes the anxiety of not knowing, intellectually, whether or not one has done the right thing. Acknowledging that there are different 'right' answers is perhaps the single most important thing that can be learnt from incorporating ethical thinking into the education of health professionals. It is surely the understanding of the point that assuming different moral standpoints can lead to different outcomes which, nevertheless can be logically defended, that can reduce the internal stress in the life of a midwife when she makes a difficult moral decision. Likewise if she can understand the priorities and focus of her clients and employers, she can accept that some degree of disharmony is inevitable.

The uses of codes generally

Professional codes have quite a variety of uses. They are acknowledged (Harris, 1989) as a mark of a profession. A little cynically, some bodies are accused of adopting a code of practice in order to become professions. In part this is offered as an explanation for the great increase in numbers of codes in existence at the present time. It surely is not the case that the mere adoption of a code can by itself constitute a body of a particular kind of workers into a profession. It may be that a body of workers, for example bankers, adopts a code as a visible sign that it is taking seriously criticism of the moral conduct of its members and to avoid the likelihood that more detailed external or statutory regulation of conduct will be imposed. This would still be a rather negative aspect of a code and one which rather definitely places the main function of codes on the side of discipline. In such a picture the code would be regarded at best as a necessary evil but at worst a 'watchdog' and as such an unwelcome source of constraint.

More purposefully, the code is used by self-governing professional bodies (another important feature of professions) to communicate their requirements to their members. If someone is not prepared to abide by 'the rules' of the profession, then membership of that body is forfeited. If there can be shown to be good reasons for being a member of a professional body, then this sort of function may contain the beginnings at least of a positive relationship between the code and the members of that particular professional body. It would seem essential if the code is to make any real contribution towards the moral conduct of a group, that it should be viewed in a positive rather than in a fearful or negative way. There is surely something unhealthy and counterproductive about moral rules being imposed and enforced in an atmosphere of oppressive power and/or fear. In the view of this author such an atmosphere is more appropriate to law enforcement than to moral guidelines.

The code in its most useful function has the potential to advise, even encourage members to behave in a moral way, over and above what they are legally obliged to do. If moral behaviour is no better than legal behaviour, there seems little point in talking about codes or professionalism at all. Indeed, it can be said that it is a great failing of many so-called codes of ethics or practice that they merely set out what an employer or employee is legally obliged to do. Such a code could surely not defend itself against an accusation that it was a mere sham, a cosmetic marketing of assumed virtue. For a code to succeed as a moral document it must somehow advise and support its readers to behave in a way which the professional body, at least, will recognize as good behaviour. In real terms it is unlikely that this can be achieved by a written code alone and it seems more likely that the code will be successful in its aim if combined with effective moral education. Such education would, in the writer's view, have two main functions: first, to discuss the intrinsic values of the profession and second, to learn and understand how these are reflected in the code. Such a process would go a long way towards getting over the problem that moral imperatives, which comprise the code (Harris, 1994) are imposed on members rather than individually decided upon. In this way the values can at least be individually ratified. In order to do this, case studies and examples of how ethical issues are manifested in the particular profession can be looked at (Hunt, 1994). In this way a midwife will have a realistic chance of knowing what sort of a behaviour would be morally acceptable within the prescripts of the code and the professional body. If codes are to be a part of the way a profession operates, then it must surely be important for them to operate in as positive a way as possible.

The use of the code of conduct in midwifery: making friends with the code

The phrase 'making friends with the code' is chosen as part of the search for a positive use of the code in the working life of the midwife. This task is as important for the UKCC as it is for the individual midwife. At a time when the practice of midwifery is likely to undergo widespread change, in attitude as well as conduct, particularly regarding the possible implementation of recommendations from *Midwives and Changing Childbirth* (Walton and Hamilton, 1995), the UKCC is especially charged with the duty of supporting midwives in their practice as well as governing them. The code and various other booklets produced by the UKCC, are the most convenient means whereby the UKCC can offer and provide support to midwives in their individual practice. However, there is very little evidence in the code that the opportunity of providing this support is being taken. Ethical training will be given by a great variety of institutions and people in a great variety of ways, but the code is the same for everyone, and as such it is the obvious vehicle for the profession to use. For example it might be helpful if the code contained some guidance as to what priority should be given to the various sets of rules that apply to midwives' practice.

The professional body would be well advised to consider the effect on their authority of a clause in a contract of employment. By putting a contractual obligation in the employment contract the employee may be under a stronger obligation (one that is more readily enforceable) to abide by the letter of their contract.

I have spoken at some length about the intrinsic values of different professions and that in any multidisciplinary scenario moral action is likely to produce tensions and dilemmas. It would be helpful if the UKCC and any ethical training approved by them could have regard to the 'pecking order' that should be applied to resolve disputes. It may be appropriate in team practice for the decision of the lead professional to be binding. Unless these issues are addressed the potential for smooth-running multiprofessional practice will be undermined. Guidance concerning disputes with management should also be considered. However, guidelines should not be used, by anyone, as a means of undermining the professional identity or value of another group. By following any guidelines prepared by the UKCC, it should be understood that those professionals trust the UKCC to 'fight their corner' on wider fronts. Local level guidelines for dispute resolution should help take some of the strain out of the working life of ever increasingly burdened midwives.

This public dimension is only one aspect of the relationship between individual practitioner and the professional body. Another important feature of professions in general is that they are empowered to police themselves (Harris, 1989). Thus when we 'make friends with the code' we must understand disciplinary matters. Sometimes the ethical aspects of good practice can be obscured by the minutiae of procedures and specific treatments; for instance, I have already mentioned that it is a common belief that a midwife very often makes a moral decision through 'gut reaction'. In terms of the relationship enjoyed between the individual practitioner and the professional body this tendency can be destructive. The danger to the practitioner involves the notes that she will, or more importantly, will not be keeping. In a court of law or a disciplinary hearing the midwife will be judged on her records. This gut reaction will be inadmissible as evidence in her defence. This whole process of moral discourse needs to be brought to the foreground of practice. If not, the practice notes will tell only a part of the story. It is clear from the list of disciplinary proceedings where practitioners are not struck off, in relation to section seven of the UKCC booklet on complaints procedure, that the UKCC want to be made aware of what thinking processes went on. The implication is, though it does not say so and should in no way be taken for granted, that provided that the tribunal is satisfied there was, for example, an absence of malice, penalties for wrong doing will not be so severe.

Ethical training in decision-making

Enough of theorizing, the ultimate question must now be faced. How is a decision made ethically? This question must be distinguished from, 'what is it ethical to do?'

It has been acknowledged that there may well be tension between the values of a midwife as an individual and the values that the profession itself seeks to impose. It has also been pointed out that even within the profession itself, the values reflected in the code come both from the practising midwives and in part from some external, perhaps, 'ideal' source. If training in ethics is to be successful, it must enable the professional to unravel these inconsistencies with a view to changing the code. The ability to influence the content of a new code will be dependent on a large number of contingencies. For example, the degree of consultation that takes place when a new code is made, economic constraints on what a midwife can herself achieve and/or what the professional body is able or willing to do. Nevertheless, even though the process may seem overly theoretical or idealistic, it is believed that there is point in the endeavour.

It will first be necessary to identify what inconsistencies may exist. This will involve some discussion of terms. While it might be assumed that all midwives want to be beneficent it cannot be assumed that each will think the same course of action will promote the client's welfare. 'Good practice' is not an absolute whereby it is always good to do the same thing. On the contrary what it means in terms of action is constantly changing. It varies for a great variety of reasons from scientific discoveries, changes in management, changes in government, ideas and practices imported from other countries and cultures which can range from deep and very significant reasons to mere fashion. All of these reasons can be factors in what constitutes good practice. How then can broad-ranging, often very general, theories of what might be good in the world possibly be helpful in deciding whether to squat or lie down to give birth?

Opinion as well as belief informs the way most of us make decisions. What ethics attempts to do is to help us to identify why we do something or, more pointedly, why we think that it is good to do a certain thing and then the practicalities of what action and how it is to be carried out can be addressed.

The tensions and differences that exist between our private and our public values, loosely categorized as 'home' and 'work' values, will almost certainly be fed by significant prejudices. These may be small or large, harmful or petty but they should be identified and acknowledged. Unless they are acknowledged consciously they cannot be ascribed a true weighting as to their influence on the way we think and why we might favour one practice or another.

Learning how to question in this way helps one to make decisions ethically. In this honest and open atmosphere of analysis, it is logical to test out whether one theory or another will be most appropriate. While in the discussion about whether or not codes were completely based on Kantian ethics, they were 'allowed' to retain that title although they did not fit exactly with Kant's philosophy, it should be noted that if the whole of a theory is not accepted then strictly speaking, the theory must be rejected in its entirety. In practice though there are many more philosophies than there are complete theories. Professional life is certainly influenced as much by utilitarianism as by Kant, as it takes place in a society that is largely influenced by utilitarianism.

In short the picture is a complex one but the struggle to find out more is a worthy one. Above all ethics is about the process rather than the outcome. No moral philosopher, however, would take up the challenge unless they were in some way concerned with finding the good. By definition that, too, is what the professional wants. Let ethics help the endeavour.

Conclusion

When faced with a series of options a decision must be made. Surely the more comfortable a professional is with the processes of logical thinking and the various theories that are available, the easier that decision will be. It is still the case at law that negligence will not usually be found in a case where a professional has made an 'honest mistake'. Although negligence can be committed by act or omission, provided that the midwife has taken account of all the circumstances, which of course includes knowledge of what is accepted as good practice and reflectively come to a decision in good faith, it would be very hard for a court of law, or anybody else, to find her culpable. It is to help her in that process that ethical training is important. To make ethics and philosophy understandable to the midwife cannot fail to be beneficial.

I have discussed the role of professions and considered what 'good' would mean in terms of the profession of midwifery. The role of the professional body has been shown as central to professional life. The professional code is the most convenient vehicle of communication between that body and the midwife. The success of the relationship depends, in moral terms, on the two-way nature of the duties of care. It is not enough for the UKCC to set standards and exercise a disciplinary function over (*inter alia*) midwives. They must support and fight for their members on the broad arena in order to deserve their moral, not just legal, allegiance.

References

Airaksinen, T. (1994). Service and science in professional life. In *Ethics and the Professions* (R. Chadwick, ed.), pp. 1–13, Avebury.

Chadwick, R. (ed.) (1994). *Ethics and the Professions*. Avebury.

Edgar, E. (1994). The value of codes of conduct. In *Ethical Issues in Nursing* (G. Hunt, ed.), pp. 148–63, Routledge.

Francome, C., Savage, W., Churchill, H. and Lewison, H. (1993). *Caesarean Birth in Britain*. Middlesex University Press.

Harris, N. (1989). *Professional Codes of Conduct in the United Kingdom: a Directory*. Mansell.

Harris, N. (1994). Professional Codes and Kantian duties. In *Ethics and the Professions* (R. Chadwick, ed.), pp. 104–15, Avebury.

Hunt, G. (ed.) (1994). *Ethical Issues in Nursing*. Routledge.

Hutchinson, D. S. (1995). Ethics. In *The Cambridge Companion to Aristotle* (J. Barnes, ed.), pp. 195–232, Cambridge University Press.

Koehn, D. (1994). *The Ground of Professional Ethics*. Routledge.

Pritchard, J. Acting professionally: Something that business organisations and individuals both desire? In *Ethical Issues in Business* (P. Davies, ed.) Routledge (in press).

Thomson, J. A. K. (translation). (1953). *The Ethics of Aristotle*. Penguin Books.

Tur, R. (1994). Accountability and lawyers. In *Ethics and the Professions* (R. Chadwick, ed.), pp. 58–87, Avebury.

Walton, I. and Hamilton, M. (1995). *Midwives and Changing Childbirth*. Books for Midwives Press Ltd.

Chapter 12

Midwifery autonomy and the code of professional conduct: An unethical combination

Rachel Clarke

The cruellest lies are often told in silence (Robert Louis Stevenson).

Introduction

Deep in the psyche of midwifery lies the myth of the independent, autonomous practitioner. Belief in this myth is the result of a fractured reflection of midwifery's perception of itself which is rarely, if ever, questioned by midwives. Can midwives identify from whom or what they are independent? Can they demonstrate professional autonomy in an environment beset with policies, protocols and contractual obligations where their practice is as confined as the women they attend? The contrast between the myth of professional freedom and the observed control of midwives by the state, through employers and medicine, exposes the fallibility of the midwife's beliefs about her autonomous status in 20th-century child-bearing.

Despite the recommendations of *Changing Childbirth* (Department of Health, 1993), the midwife is unlikely to achieve the status of an autonomous provider of maternity care without the aid of political and legal intervention. Present government policy is to leave the implementation of the recommendations to local health service trusts, rather than intervene on a political or legislative level to overcome medicine's monopoly of maternity care.

This situation reflects the flaws in the 1902 Midwives Act, which acknowledged the practitioner status of midwives, but failed to give them self regulation, that is, the right to define the scope of their professional authority and sphere of control. The rival profession of medicine was to have 'a dominant voice in their government' (Donnison, 1988). Over the last 30 years the medicalization of child-bearing and the close association of midwifery with obstetrics have led to the obstetrician being acknowledged as the standard setter for midwifery practice. In the legal debate over the scope of practice it remains to be seen if traditional midwifery would be recognized by the courts as being superior to scientific biomedical obstetrics. Therefore, authentic professional autonomy has not been, and is unlikely to be, realistically within reach.

Until relatively recently midwifery autonomy was not an issue. Belief by midwives in its existence was harmless enough and it was of little consequence to obstetricians, who simply smiled behind the backs of midwives and continued to control child-bearing events from conception to birth. However, two events served to highlight the tension between the real and imagined nature of professional autonomy for midwives. The first was the 1979 Nurses, Midwives and Health Visitors Act, which established the United Kingdom Central Council (UKCC) as the statutory regulatory body for nurses, midwives and health visitors (which became fully functional in 1983). The second occurred in 1988 when a midwife in private practice, Jilly Rosser, was struck off the register by the UKCC for professional misconduct.

As part of its statutory duty to safeguard the public interest, establish and improve standards of training and professional conduct for nursing and midwifery, the UKCC published the Code of Professional Conduct (UKCC, 1992). This document introduced the professions to the concept of individual professional and moral accountability and the disciplinary framework which would be responsible for regulating professional conduct.

The Code is representative of a dimension of ethics known as prescriptive ethics, an approach which gives rise to policies, guidelines and codes of conduct/practice in an attempt to establish what one ought or ought not to do in practice. Such an approach further supposes that there is a definitive response to a situation and a definitive answer to a dilemma (see Chapter 11). In this respect the Code has not moved away from the historical legacy of strictly regulating the activities of nurses and midwives. In the past these professions have been overly concerned with attempting to standardize behaviour by using rules to prescribe right and wrong actions, rather than concentrating their efforts on identifying the dynamic nature of practice and the moral dimension of caring as a skilled, therapeutic activity. The Code of Professional Conduct exhibits what can only be called professional schizophrenia, for it purports to be a document of principles, open to interpretation by informed, autonomous practitioners, when in truth it affirms the tradition of maintaining the homogeneous predictability of nursing/midwifery.

Underlying the assumption that practitioners are able to exercise professional and moral autonomy unfettered by the constraints of their employers and medical practitioners is a disregard for the true status of nurses and midwives as employees of the NHS. The professional mandate of the Code, arising from the statutory responsibility of the UKCC, is to safeguard, promote and protect the interests of patients at all times. This is a somewhat problematic mandate, given the restrictive nature of the role of nurses and midwives in the NHS.

In this chapter I argue that the UKCC is profoundly unjust in expecting midwives to practise autonomously, as required by the Code of Professional Conduct. Further, the Code is fundamentally flawed and therefore unethical for the following reason – it is based on the unwarranted assumption that midwives are autonomous practitioners professionally, clinically and morally.

Professional, clinical and moral autonomy are prerequisites for interpreting and following the Code's guidelines. Further, in order for midwives to be accountable they must be autonomous and it is on this basis that the UKCC carries out its regulatory function of holding midwives accountable to the public in a fair and just manner. The fact that professional, clinical and moral accountability are not key features of midwifery practice casts grave doubts upon the UKCC's ability to perform this function ethically.

Outline of the Code

The Code was imposed upon the workforce without consultation. Reg Pyne, the assistant registrar for standards and ethics at the UKCC when the Code was first published, said that, 'there was no reason for the

UKCC to be shy nor hesitant in its advice, nor did it have to dilute what is expected from practitioners or hold back from stating its view of the ideal' (Pyne, 1987). He also admitted that the purpose behind the Code was, 'to convert the profession from one that has seen good conduct as being compliant and submissive, to a profession that sees it as being more assertive and questioning' (Carlisle, 1989). However, on the methods by which the professions of nursing and midwifery would be converted to these new values, the UKCC remained silent.

There is little evidence to support claims by the UKCC that the Code is a source of empowerment to practitioners and this has led to widespread criticism of the Code. Tadd (1994) puts forward the notion that the Code is simply an exercise in tokenism and questions whether the Code has made any difference to the moral climate of nursing and midwifery. Considering the rigid, policy-driven working structure experienced by midwives, the answer to the question is likely to be 'No'.

The Code is presented in terms of abstract concepts and ambiguous statements, which are difficult to interpret, yet appear deceptively simple to the unwary; for example, the first paragraph states that each practitioner must 'act always in such a manner as to promote and safeguard the interests and well-being of patients and clients.' What does this really mean and how far should a midwife go to safeguard these interests?

A woman is about to undergo a planned, non-emergency Caesarean section. Once under the anaesthetic, the obstetrician invites two or three junior doctors to perform vaginal examinations on her to add to their experience. The woman has not consented to these multiple examinations. When the midwife in theatre questions the ethics of this practice she is told by the obstetrician, 'What she doesn't know can't hurt her.' The midwife knows that examinations performed without consent constitute the civil tort of battery. She also knows that they are not in the woman's best interests. What is she to do if she is to safeguard those interests? This question has professional, moral and legal dimensions.

The Code of Professional Conduct states that each nurse, midwife and health visitor shall act at all times in such a manner as to:

(1) safeguard and promote the interests of individual patients and clients;
(2) serve the interests of society;

(3) justify public trust and confidence;
(4) uphold and enhance the good standing and reputation of the professions.

In trying to decide how the midwife might act in the example above, the ambiguities of the Code become apparent. How is the midwife to safeguard and promote the interests of the patient without exposing the unethical and illegal practice of the obstetrician? How can public trust and confidence be justified if midwives are seen to be involved in the exposure of the injustices of medicine? The result would be professionally divisive and place the midwife in jeopardy of losing her job.

Due to its deceptive simplicity the moral nature of the Code has remained invisible to the majority of practitioners and so too have the dangers arising from simplistic interpretations, making the Code a dangerous document in the hands of the morally and politically naive. How are the *interests* of any patient to be defined and identified? What would happen if the midwife's interpretation of *interest* clashed with the obstetrician's interpretation? Whose definition of interests would have priority in the care of the patient? The ramifications of these demands are enormous. Not only is the practice of an individual now compared with an ideal, the individual is also punished for failing to live up to that ideal, despite the constraints that make that ideal impossible to achieve.

When practitioners have taken issue with the UKCC decision to strike them off the professional register and taken their cases to court, the courts have been critical of the UKCC and its idealistic expectations, in many instances ordering the UKCC to restore practitioners to the register. The attitude of the courts is that the UKCC is too punitive in its enforcement of the idealistic standards of the Code of Professional Conduct (Flint, 1989).

Midwifery practice and the concept of autonomy

While there is little evidence to support the midwife's claim to autonomy, there is considerable evidence to undermine it. Midwifery research has given us significant insights into the real nature of present-day practice that includes apathy, inertia and lack of control surrounding the exercising of clinical judgement and decision making. These characteristics are a legacy of midwifery's modern development and it is here that we find the basis for midwifery dependency.

The impact of the 1902 Midwives Act

The history of midwifery and women healers has been chronicled by many able authors (Donnison, 1988; Achterberg, 1991; Garcia *et al.*, 1990), all of whom capture the difficulties, the attitudes and the aspirations of the rival occupations of midwifery and obstetrics, charting the decline of the midwife and her transformation into obstetric assistant during the 20th century.

The 1902 Midwives Act was a critical turning point for midwifery. It offered education, state registration and the prospect of respectability. It was welcomed with great warmth and enthusiasm by the Midwives Institute (first formed in 1880 as the Matron's Aid Society and now the Royal College of Midwives), whose primary aim was to raise the status of the occupation in order to attract middle-class women into the profession and improve standards, thereby offering greater protection for women in childbirth from incompetent midwives. There was, however, a price to be paid. In return for the continued tenure of midwifery, midwives not only had to accept a restricted sphere of practice which would be defined by medical men, they also had to surrender their autonomy.

The Central Midwives Board, created by the 1902 Act to regulate the education, training and registration of midwives, had no requirement to include midwives in its membership. Furthermore, when this was finally granted in 1920, it was statutorily forbidden for midwives to be in a majority. Medical practitioners had reason to be pleased: having control of midwifery education and practice through their influence on the Central Midwives Board would ensure that midwives stayed in their lowly and proper place, 'what you want to educate midwives for is for them to know their own ignorance, that is really the one great object in educating midwives' (Select Committee on Midwives' Registration, 1892, cited in Witz, 1988).

Medical practitioners had drawn clear lines between what was midwives' work and what was doctors' work. The Midwives Institute accepted the division, making it quite clear they had every intention of working in harmony with doctors. Their betrayal of midwifery struck the most damaging blow to the achievement of full professional status. When the 1902 Act was passed, midwifery became a semi-profession and one subservient to medicine.

The 1902 Act preserved the midwife in name, but reduced her competence and sphere of practice. She was left with the relatively unskilled role of attending at normal births (see Chapter 5), and the new rules made sure she called the doctor for any deviation or face the possibility of losing her registration. Witz (1988) describes the method used to quell midwifery independence as a gendered strategy of de-skilling, demarcation and incorporation. It was spectacularly successful, for not only did midwives allow themselves to be manipulated into a position of subservience in 1902, they have never, at any time later, made any attempt to overthrow the oppressive influence of obstetrics. Obstetrics has continued to incorporate normal, healthy pregnant women into the medical domain and establish its credibility with the public by extolling the virtues of the scientific application of technology to achieve a safe birth.

The remainder of the 20th century has seen a continued decline in midwifery skills and midwifery control in direct proportion to the growth of interventionist obstetrics and its philosophy that birth is only normal in retrospect. The effects of the decline in traditional midwifery skills and confidence will be of particular concern in the near future. As a result of *Changing Childbirth* (Department of Health, 1993), which appears to endorse freedom of choice by the consumer and a higher profile for midwives as the lead professional in the care of healthy child-bearing women, many midwives may now feel unprepared and unwilling to accept this proposed level of responsibility.

Following the 1979 Nurses, Midwives and Health Visitors Act, the UKCC took control of the education of nurses and midwives, restructuring it so that the medical influence was reduced. Nevertheless, in midwifery the medical obstetric influence endures through its emphasis on the pathology of child-bearing and by the relentless, insidious destruction of traditional midwifery knowledge. Midwifery endorses this by default in approving obstetric units as suitable training establishments in which to learn midwifery. This legacy of subservience and powerlessness is responsible for the absence of professional, clinical and moral autonomy of midwives.

Autonomy and midwifery: some evidence

According to John Harris (1992), 'people are said to be autonomous to the extent to which they are able to control their own lives, and to some extent their own destiny, by the exercise of their own faculties.' Autonomy is not a commodity. It cannot be bought or sold or collected piecemeal. It is a characteristic of individuals who are able to direct their lives according to their own desires. For a professional group, autonomy is expressed in the way it defines and directs its own sphere of business/practice, provides appropriate education/training and monitors its members by a process of internal regulation without interference from others. Having endured control by the Central Midwives Board which lacked adequate midwifery representation, midwifery now endures control by the UKCC, which tends to include midwives under the generic term *nurses* and limits the influence of the Midwifery Committees set up to protect professional interests.

Significantly, the role of midwives continues to be defined by medical personnel and employers. Beauchamp and Childress (1994) comment that autonomy must include 'personal rule of the self free from controlling interferences by others.' Nevertheless, controlling interferences continue to undermine the midwife's opportunities to learn, achieve and exercise her full professional role. Harris cites four defects which can diminish autonomy, one of which is particularly useful when examining midwifery autonomy: 'defects in the individual's ability to control either her desires or her actions, or both' (Harris, 1992).

The changes in the midwife's role and responsibilities brought about by the increased medicalization and hospitalization of birth further restricted the boundaries of her role, influenced the way she made decisions in the execution of her role and changed the way she perceived her role *vis-à-vis* that of the doctor. Influences on the education and training of midwives have altered the learning experience, so that they have come to regard obstetric values and practices as representative of midwifery. As a result of these changes there are four areas of critical significance where there are serious defects in control: clinical practice, the clinical learning environment, ownership of the patient (accountability) and the exercise of clinical judgement. These will be considered in turn.

Clinical practice

The work of Robinson *et al.* (1983) has illustrated the lack of control the midwife has over her work. They have made the revealing observation that midwives frequently overestimate the extent to which they use their clinical judgement and seriously underestimate the extent to which obstetric policies exert control over their decisions. This is particularly evident when caring for women in labour. Robinson and her colleagues are not alone in making these observations; Henderson (1984), Garcia *et al.* (1985) and Garcia and Garforth (1991) have all demonstrated similar findings regarding some of the key areas of management of women in labour; for example, performing vaginal examinations; deciding to rupture the membranes; and deciding to use electronic fetal monitoring.

The practice of performing four-hourly vaginal examinations is a particularly interesting one, for no work has been done to support the value of such a regimen. Its purpose is to produce conformance to the obstetric partogram (a graph on which all labour events are charted), in order to give an illustrated progress report on labour. In performing this four-hourly procedure, which is unnecessary, invasive and unevaluated, midwives reveal a marked lack of professional and clinical autonomy. It is extremely doubtful that midwives would now be willing to forgo the routine four-hourly vaginal examination in favour of skilled abdominal assessment, due to the lack of skill and confidence induced by exposure to obstetric influence and the general fear of litigation.

One of the disturbing features of Robinson's study (Robinson *et al.*, 1983) was the degree of acquiescence that midwives demonstrated to doctors taking over completely, or replicating the most basic aspects of their role. The data showed a substantial number of midwives never had an opportunity to rely entirely on their own skills and judgements in assessing the course of pregnancy, because the medical staff took over this responsibility. Yet this is an aspect of practice that is fundamental, not only to the midwife's role but to her very existence! In the key area of abdominal examination, almost all midwives in the study felt that this was a task appropriate for the midwife, yet almost all the hospital midwives and two-thirds of community midwives worked in situations where the doctor carried out this examination and, despite this, an astonishing 60% of hospital midwives and 72% of community midwives felt this division of responsibility was about right (Robinson *et al.*, 1983).

Despite the reassuring confirmation that the midwife is the person who delivers over 70% of babies, it is optimistic to take this as an indicator of autonomy. Even here, management of key areas such as the length of the second stage of labour and the method of delivery of the placenta and membranes are controlled by arbitrary, obstetrically derived time limits and methodology (see Chapter 5). Evidence of the erosion of midwifery skills arising from the medicalization of labour became evident in the Bristol Third Stage Trial, a research study which set out to compare outcomes of different management approaches to the third stage of labour (Inch, 1990). The declaration that the trial was invalid was due, in part, to the lack of knowledge and skill of the midwives who were assigned to conduct normal, physiological delivery of placenta and membranes. In short, they did not know how. Their training as students and their practice as qualified midwives had never enabled them to gain expertise in traditional midwifery skills, one of which is the management of a completely physiological delivery of placenta and membranes.

Since the work of Robinson, Golden and Bradley, 1983 (Robinson *et al.*, 1983) there has been no similar study to re-assess the midwife's role in the UK, but there is little cause to suppose any fundamental change has occurred. Since the publication of *Changing Childbirth* (Department of Health, 1993), the Royal College of Obstetricians and Gynaecologists has made it clear that its members are opposed to the proposed changes, which include making the midwife the lead professional in the care of normal, healthy women. They want the term 'lead professional' replaced by 'link professional'. They question the reduced input from obstetricians in the care of normal women (which they say is unacceptable) and they express the fear (somewhat tongue-in-cheek?) that the midwife may become isolated if she becomes an independent practitioner (Dunlop, 1993). The root of this conflict lies in delineating professional power and obstetricians will go to great lengths to maintain the status quo. It does not augur well. The midwife's role will not change significantly whilst obstetricians continue to exert control over child-bearing events.

The effects of the learning environment

Training schools for midwives must be approved by the appropriate National Board (part of the statutory structures set up by the 1979 Act to assist the UKCC). It is not just the educational establishment that must be approved; the obstetric unit in which students gain their practical experience must also be approved.

The irony is that midwives so lack control over their own education that they give approval to obstetric units as suitable places to learn normal, traditional midwifery skills. These are the very places where such experience is either unavailable or available so infrequently that no student or midwife could accumulate sufficient experience to claim that she was an expert in normal (physiological) child-bearing events. In obstetric units students of midwifery find it impossible to witness 10 deliveries of women whose labours were completely physiological, followed by their supervised personal management of 40 further cases, also completely physiological. It is not surprising that the work of Robinson *et al.* (1983) and the results of the Bristol trial demonstrated such a marked and fundamental shift in the knowledge and skills of midwives. If midwifery approves the placing of students in obstetric units where what they learn is obstetrically oriented, it must accept responsibility for the outcome: midwives who are ill-prepared and reluctant to accept the validity of midwife-led, low-technology, low intervention care outside of the confines of a medically oriented unit. The lack of control in this key area of midwifery is crucial to understanding why midwives are generally unwilling and unable to take control of the management of child-bearing women.

Ownership of the patient and accountability

There is a third, equally critical area, where midwives exhibit lack of control. The Code's foremost principle is the *primacy of the patient* and the practitioner is required to 'safeguard and protect the interests of individual patients and clients.' Safeguarding these interests, which are left to the practitioner to discern, frequently brings the individual into conflict with medical staff and employers. The now famous case of Graham Pink, the nurse who tried desperately in his patients' best interests to use the Code to draw attention to gross understaffing which, he said resulted in poor patient care, graphically illustrated to nurses and midwives their isolated and helpless status. Whilst the investigating committee of the English National Board for Nursing, Midwifery and Health Visiting decided not to refer Mr Pink's case to the UKCC, his employers found him guilty of gross professional misconduct, a situation in which the UKCC was unable to intervene effectively (Carlisle and Hempel, 1991). Whistle-blowing, especially by nursing staff, has never been popular in the NHS but this is exactly what practitioners are required to do in their patients' best interests, regardless of the consequences for the individual practitioners concerned. Consider the following example based on real events.

A consultant obstetrician, who is fervently anti-abortion, nevertheless offers amniocentesis to a woman. During the procedure, he deliberately draws off an insufficient amount of liquor to enable the laboratory staff to perform the tests that will determine possible abnormality of the fetus. The midwife knows what he has done and she has seen him do this on every other occasion she has assisted him at the procedure. By the time the woman returns for her results it is too late for a repeat test. The midwife knows that it is a ploy on his part to avoid the possibility of termination should there be an abnormality of the developing fetus.

The Code requires this midwife to act in a way that safeguards and protects the patient's best interests. There are two issues here: first, the midwife does not have a patient, the patient *belongs* to the consultant who alone has the legitimate authority to diagnose, treat and discharge the patient. How can the midwife act in the patient's best interests when, in effect, she has no patient and no authority to act on her behalf? Second, the UKCC has burdened practitioners with the *moral* ownership of patients and demands that they carry *moral responsibility* for them. If the midwife tells the woman what has happened, she might choose to go elsewhere for her antenatal care and she might also complain loudly about the reason why. The midwife puts herself at risk of being charged with gross professional misconduct by her employer and she is likely to be dismissed for lowering the integrity of the medical staff in the eyes of the patient.

There are other examples that exemplify the power differential between medical staff and midwives. When a woman is pregnant with twins and one of them has a condition that is incompatible with life, it is the doctor alone who has the power to decide if the woman is not to be told. The midwife must continue to provide midwifery care within this wall of silence. Authentic midwifery has become invisible within obstetrics and she is permitted only to provide midwifery care *as it is defined by obstetrics*, that is, carry out those routine observations and monitoring tasks that do not require, and indeed prevent, the establishment of professional intimacy and responsibility. Even if the midwife believes she has a moral duty to inform the woman of the situation she dare not do so; the doctor's decision is final and the midwife does not have the authority to overturn the clinical judgement of the doctor (Dimond, 1990).

Evidence of defects in control continues to be a feature of the institution of midwifery and of midwifery practice and seriously undermines the claim that midwives are professionally autonomous. The evidence also casts doubt on the assumption of the UKCC that midwives have the professional, clinical and moral autonomy necessary to practise as directed by the Code of Professional Conduct.

Clinical judgement and the case of Jilly Rosser

In 1988 when Jilly Rosser was struck off the register by the UKCC, the problematic nature of midwifery autonomy and the idealistic nature of the UKCC's expectations of midwives became manifest.

Jilly Rosser was found guilty of professional misconduct and removed from the register. The evidence for misconduct included criticism of Rosser's record keeping and the decision to transfer her patient (who was haemorrhaging, following a birth at home) to hospital in her own car rather than wait for the emergency services to arrive.

In response to the charge about her records, Rosser claimed that her records were made as the situation permitted, in accord with Rule 42 of the Midwives Rules, which among other things states that records will be made 'as contemporaneously as is reasonable' (UKCC, 1993). In response to the second charge regarding the use of her own car to transport the patient to hospital, Rosser claimed that her professional knowledge and experience of the poor performance of the emergency services in responding to calls enabled her to predict with a high degree of certainty that her patient's condition would deteriorate significantly if she waited for them to arrive. With this local knowledge and her midwifery experience, Rosser arrived at a clinical decision which she believed best served her patient's interests.

Rosser's clinical decision was not accepted by the Professional Conduct Committee of the UKCC who declared her guilty of professional misconduct and removed her name from the register. Rosser was unhappy with this judgement and took the case to the High Court. It was hoped that the judge, Lord Justice Watkins, would interpret the meaning of misconduct but his judgement was not heard because the UKCC, in what Flint (1989) calls a 'face-saving exercise', conceded the case and withdrew. Rosser was allowed her appeal and the UKCC was ordered to reinstate her on the register.

During the case, Lord Justice Watkins questioned the unrealistic expectations of the UKCC regarding midwives' capabilities. It was his opinion that Rosser's records were satisfactory up until the time of the emergency but, he pointed out, she would then have been engaged in examining her patient, contacting the patient's general practitioner and arranging for her transfer to hospital. The barrister acting for the UKCC claimed that Rosser should have been jotting down notes whilst holding the patient's hand, to which Lord Justice Watkins replied, 'she would have to be a first class juggler.' Lord Justice Watkins went on to say that he found the charge against Rosser taking the patient to hospital in her own car to be *perverse* and asked the UKCC's barrister if Rosser would be in the same situation if she had passively waited for the emergency services to arrive. This question was never answered.

In the absence of any statement from the UKCC clarifying the exact nature of Rosser's misconduct, it is disturbing to consider that the motives of the UKCC might have been more to quell midwifery independence than to protect the public from what it would have us believe was an unsafe practitioner. Significantly, the law did not find any aspect of Rosser's practice unusual or unsafe. Rosser had to make a decision about what action on her part might best safeguard and promote her patient's best interests in accord with the Code of Professional Conduct. With regard to the performance of the emergency services, would it have been in her patient's best interests to wait and bleed, perhaps to death, or was it in her best interests to be transported to hospital by any means available and as quickly as possible in order to safeguard her life? After all, staying alive is surely in her best interests? Reflecting on the words of Reg Pyne (1987) that the UKCC wanted to see a profession that was assertive and questioning and one which would act according to the Code, it is impossible to imagine how practitioners might aspire to this without exercising clinical judgement.

Clinical judgement is not definitive; it cannot be written down as an action plan for others to follow. It varies according to the situation and people involved and is a unique combination of the practitioner's responses to them. In the same way, the Code is not written in a definitive manner but in principles and concepts for the practitioner to interpret. If the UKCC wishes practitioners to interpret and act upon those principles, why did it punish Jilly Rosser for doing exactly that? Could it be that the ulterior motive of the UKCC was to use Rosser as a warning to other midwives who might be foolish enough to disturb the balance of power between doctors and other subordinate practitioners?

Maintaining midwives' lack of autonomy

Let us suppose that midwives were to be granted the same legitimate authority as the medical specialists, making clinical decisions and acting with complete professional autonomy. In the present structure of the health service this hypothetical situation of two equally autonomous practitioners who hold opposing ideologies about childbearing and who both have access to the pregnant woman makes it obvious that the relative stability would disintegrate. The pregnant woman would be a pawn between midwife and obstetrician who would vie for control of her. It would be impossible for these two very different practitioners to exist with equality, claiming ownership of child-bearing women. Is it possible that the UKCC was seeking to maintain this equilibrium?

Conclusion

In considering justice, the UKCC ought to explain to midwives how it justifies the imposition of the Code's principles upon them in an environment where the employers prohibit their freedom to act on them. The UKCC has no place in the legal contract between employer and employee. It is an uninvited third party whose values and professional mandate have little relevance to employers of midwives. Although it is acceptable to describe a future vision of midwifery as an autonomous profession and able to exercise clinical freedom, it is not acceptable to expect midwives to act as if that future vision were already reality, while judging them by the standards of today. Unacceptable as it might sound, midwives might be best advised to ignore patients' best interests in order to safeguard their own. It cannot be right in any sense that midwives become martyrs on behalf of their patients.

It is clear that professional, clinical and moral autonomy continue to elude the profession of midwifery. Without autonomy, the professional accountability of midwives remains problematical and the Code of Professional Conduct is an unsavoury reminder of the failure of the UKCC to empower its members.

References

Achterberg, J. (1991). *Woman as Healer*. Rider.

Beauchamp, T. L. and Childress, J. F. (1994). *Principles of Bio-medical Ethics*. Oxford University Press.

Carlisle, D. (1989). Silence is not golden. *Nursing Times*, **85** (36), p. 19.

Carlisle, D. and Hempel, S. (1991). Conduct Unbecoming? *Nursing Times*, **87** (30), p. 18.

Department of Health Expert Maternity Group (1993). *Changing Childbirth, Report of the Expert Maternity Group*. (The Cumberledge Report). HMSO.

Dimond, B. (1990). *Legal Aspects of Nursing*. Prentice Hall.

Donnison, J. (1988). *Midwives & Medical Men*. Historical Publications.

Dunlop, W. (1993). Changing Childbirth—Commentary II. *Br. J. Obstet. Gynaecol.*, **100**, 1072–1073.

Flint, C. (1989). A matter of judgement. *Nursing Times*, **85**, (12), p. 19.

Garcia, J. and Garforth, S. (1991). Midwifery policies and policymaking. In *Midwives, Research & Childbirth* (S. Robinson and A. Thomson, eds) vol. II, Chapman and Hall.

Garcia, J., Garforth, S. and Ayers, S. (1985). Midwives confined?: labour ward policies and routines. In *Research & the Midwife Conference Proceedings 1985*. Nursing Education Research Unit, Kings College, London University.

Garcia, J., Kilpatrick, R. and Richards, R. (1990). *The Politics of Maternity Care*. Clarendon Paperbacks.

Harris, J. (1992). *The Value of Life: An Introduction to Medical Ethics*. Routledge.

Henderson, C. (1984). Influences and interactions surrounding the midwife's decision to rupture the membranes. In *Research & the Midwife Conference Proceedings 1984*. Nursing Education Research Unit, Kings College, London University.

Inch, S. (1990). The Bristol third stage trial. *AIMS Q. J.*, **1** (4), 8–10.

Pyne, R. (1987). A professional duty to shout. *Nursing Times*, **83** (42), 30–31.

Robinson, S., Golden, J. and Bradley, S. (1983). *A Study of the Role and Responsibilities of the Midwife*. Nursing Education Research Unit, Kings College, London University.

Tadd, V. (1994). Professional Codes: an exercise in tokenism? *Nursing Ethics*, **1** (1), 15–23.

UKCC. (1992). *Code of Professional Conduct*.

UKCC. (1993). *Midwives Rules*.

Witz, A. (1988). Patriarchal relations and patterns of sex segregation. In *Gender Segregation at Work* (S. Walby, ed.) Ch. 6, Open University Press.

Chapter 13

The midwife advocate

Karen Bartter

Introduction

The position of the midwife as her client's advocate is one of growing concern. While the concept and role of the advocate is not new, its application to midwifery is relatively recent and worthy of debate. Legal advocates have been in evidence since at least the beginning of the 12th century and, according to DuCann (1980), they deal in fact and are concerned with the discovery of the truth. To some extent the midwife advocate is the same. The midwife's daily duty is concerned with the application of midwifery, with her being, on a philosophical plane at least, responsible for all that happens within midwifery and concerned with the discovery of the truth of midwifery practice. Women and society surely have a right to expect this from their midwife. Indeed, now as never before within the health care services there is a growing interest in ensuring that the rights of individual patients and clients are upheld. The Patient's Charter booklet *Maternity Services* (Department of Health, 1994) lays out the broad aspects of care users should expect from those services. The common theme of this booklet and other recent publications can be seen as illustrating the increased demand for advocacy in the NHS.

How able is the midwife for this great task? How good is she at fulfilling this part of her role? Indeed, is it even appropriate for her to attempt to undertake it? The following chapter will attempt to answer these questions. It will look at the role of advocacy in midwifery. Then two main problems with the midwife as advocate will be addressed; how to ascertain the best interests of the patient and the constraints on professional practice. The chapter will address the reality of the midwife as an advocate and close with ideas for the future.

What is an advocate?

Each nurse, midwife and health visitor is charged by the UKCC with the responsibility of being an advocate for her client. She must: 'Act always in such a way as to promote and safeguard the interests and well-being of patients and clients' (UKCC, 1992). Is this too arduous a task for the midwife to undertake?

An advocate is a noble being, a courageous, honest individual who has good judgement and is sincere and tenacious to her task. Eloquent, with a good command of language, the advocate is able to put forward a case accurately and clearly but also able to hold her tongue and control her own feelings. Ever industrious and alert to promote her client's needs and wishes, she is also knowledgeable and astute enough to accept only that which she is able successfully to undertake. The advocate fights the good fight and defends the cause. DuCann (1980) says an advocate is more than just someone who has certain duties and responsibilities; there is an art of advocacy that cannot be acquired without the natural gift. The technical rules alone are useless unless the innate ability is there, although how to apply and appropriately use it must be learned, exercised and developed.

The Cassell's English Dictionary defines an advocate as: 'One who defends or promotes a cause; one who pleads a cause; an intercessor' (Hayward and Sparkes, 1968). However, this simple description belies the complexity of this role. Whose cause is being defended? The midwife must be clear on whose behalf and in whose interests she is acting. To promote a cause one must have extensive knowledge of all aspects of the situation, the history, the future and of the individuals concerned. Furthermore, to intercede one must be willing and able to take the cause to its logical conclusion, whatever the personal risks or sacrifices involved.

Tschudin (1992) states that advocacy arises out of the ethic of caring. It rests, she says, on three common elements between people in any given relationship, those of humanity, needs and rights. Humanity is the belief that each human is morally equal, even accepting that other factors about them and their lives may not be. Needs relate to the recognized basic human needs; these range from food, shelter and protection, to the higher expectations of individual expression, and ultimately to where justice and truth are exercised equally towards each and every individual. Rights, Tschudin states, relate to the access to, and the application of the above. So advocacy is not about taking over but ensuring with the patient, on an equal humanistic plane, that their needs and rights are met. Thus, power is transferred back to patients so that they may control their own affairs. Here the advocate stands alongside patients, defending them against the unjust or unwanted course and speaking up for patients who are too ill or ignorant to do this for themselves.

Marshall (1991) follows the theme of power transferral from the professional back to the patient. She defines advocacy as involving, informing, supporting and protecting clients so that they can make their own health care decisions. She goes on to say that when needed, the nurse advocate should mediate on her client's behalf. Marshall suggests that in order to do this the advocate must be knowledgeable about all aspects of the care and the situation in question. She goes on to state that the nurse is not adequately prepared for, or supported by her colleagues, to undertake this role. However, surely the acquisition of knowledge is not the responsibility of another but of the individual practitioner and who is to say that those who suggest the course of action of which the client is unsure are any more or less knowledgeable than the nurse or midwife who opposes it. In addition, it is quite likely that no health care professional (HCP) is more knowledgeable about all aspects of the personal situation of the patient than he is himself.

Duties of the midwife advocate

The legal advocate, according to DuCann (1980), has fivefold duties: to the client, to society, to self, to other colleagues and to the professions. To some extent the midwife as advocate has corresponding duties aligned to these. Certainly she has a duty to the client, having entered into a relationship with the woman based on trust. Hence, the midwife is surely morally and professionally obliged not to misplace that trust.

Her duty to society and to the general public stems from the duty she has to the client. It is likely that over 90% of the women in our society will experience the execution of the duties of a midwife at some time in their lives. This obligation to society is clearly more obvious for the midwife than for the legal advocate, where his duty to society may have a greater philosophical than actual application.

For herself, the duty of the midwife advocate may be the most complex and yet the most simplistic. It will depend on her own moral beliefs and principles and on her understanding of the role of midwife advocate. This will be considered again later in the chapter.

It is in regard to the duties to their colleagues and the profession that the common paths of the legal and midwife advocate begin to diverge. The legal advocate's immediate colleagues are other legal advocates. These, while they might interpret the letter of the law in slightly variable ways in order to press their point to the greater advantage, are generally in agreement about the principle of the law. The position for the midwife advocate may be less uniform. Indeed, some of her very close working colleagues may be in total opposition to the adversarial stance she is taking, preferring paternalism rather than advocacy. In addition, while the legal advocate is likely to respect his fellow adversary and engage with concealed relish in the well constructed and challenging battle, such an honourable contest is not in the offing for the midwife advocate. Here a historical power struggle may cloud the rational argument as the midwife and the doctor battle for control over the patient. Even when the exchange is between midwife and midwife, objective discussion based on fact and research may be interwoven with and overshadowed by a hierarchical power struggle and an insecurity born from not wanting to suffer the consequences of rocking the boat. The midwife advocate's duty to the profession is indeed complex and will be considered in more detail shortly.

In addition to DuCann's fivefold duties of the legal advocate (DuCann, 1980), the midwife advocate has also to consider the influence of the UKCC and her position as an employee. For, unlike the legal advocate, the midwife is employed by an organization which sees the needs of each individual client as only part of the total needs and responsibilities it has to consider.

Does the midwife have DuCann's innate gift of the art of advocacy and if so is she able to recognize it and to know how and when to use it? If the midwife does not possess the gift, can she learn the art of advocacy? Can she develop the skills of knowing how and when to exercise this art? The definition of advocacy has been examined and it is now necessary to consider whether such advocacy is possible in a midwifery context.

There are two problems related to this: first, how to demonstrate the best interests of the client, and second, constraints on midwifery practice. These will be dealt with in turn.

The problem of the best interests of the client

When the midwife feels obliged to defend the needs and rights of her client, to act in her client's best interests, how can she be sure that what she is taking as her client's needs and rights are actually that? This fictitious case illustrates the point.

Marie Smith lay gently propped up, alone and afraid. Thanks to the epidural the labour was barely uncomfortable, but she was trapped, with immobile useless legs, an infusion in her arm, a fine plastic tube in her back and a monitor strapped to her abdomen. She lay listening to her fetus's heartbeat.

Marie Smith had trusted the midwife.

'I'll do all I can to see that you get what you want in your labour, that you have what is best for you and your baby,' the midwife had said.

Marie Smith had wanted to be mobile and had wanted to be in control.

Midwife Phillips handed over report and care of Marie Smith to Midwife Jones for the next shift. She was pleased with herself. She had acted as advocate for Marie Smith and for her fetus. The labour was painful for the mother, so she had fetched the doctor who had given the patient an epidural. The fetus was not reacting too favourably to the induction of the labour, so she was continuously monitoring it to be sure it was all right. Her records were clear, accurate and up-to-date. Every time she had called the doctors, or reported progress to them, she had recorded and signed to that effect in the appropriate documents. Marie Smith was well hydrated, comfortable, able to watch television and summon her known named midwife at the push of a button. All she had to do was wait for the birth of her baby. Midwife Phillips had been the best possible advocate for her client. She went off duty confident in her abilities.

Yet Midwife Phillips did have nagging doubts over the case. She had to accept that her patient had said that she did not want aggressive pain control, or anything that would reduce her mobility, as she had wanted to be upright, mobile and in control. The doctor had said that it was really for the best and that women could not really be expected truly to know what they wanted when they were experiencing so much labour pain. And yet, research did suggest that mobility and support in labour could achieve as favourable an outcome for a woman and her fetus as more active and controlled management did. But no, she had not really wanted a stand-up argument with that particular doctor, especially as the patient would probably have ended up with the same final outcome whatever she had done.

Marie Smith subsequently went on to deliver a live, healthy 7 lb baby girl with minimal trauma to mother and child. After a seemingly uneventful postnatal recovery, she wrote a letter of complaint to the hospital committee.

Was Midwife Phillips engaging in the art of advocacy for her patient?

Surely every woman would want a pain-free, comfortable labour that culminated in the birth of a live, healthy baby with the minimum of trauma to both? Obviously an apparently total physical recovery for the mother, with her achieving competence in the care of herself and her baby are honourable aims for HCP to want for all women in their care. Indeed, these very ideals form the backbone of the organization, structure and delivery of midwifery care (Garrey et al., 1980; Bennett and Brown, 1989; Enkin et al., 1990; Silverton, 1993). How could any woman complain? Fulfilment of these aims reduces morbidity and mortality for women and their babies, creates satisfaction for consumers and carers alike and is an excellent cost-effective tactic when considering minimum total expenditure for optimum output gains. That is, if women have more pain in labour, for example, they require more labour-intensive midwifery input, have the potential for more operative deliveries, which may necessitate a longer in-patient hospital stay and have babies which may not be in optimum health. All of which require more specialist input and have the potential for more minor or major postnatal recovery problems, and if women are ineffective at self and baby care, this all equals an increased expenditure for the same number of deliveries.

It must be made quite clear that there is no suggestion that a woman or the professional serving her would actively seek any one scenario for care over another. To make such a suggestion would be as equally judgemental, prejudiced and paternalistic as to suggest that every woman wants *exactly* the same outcome as the next for *her* childbirth experience. But certainly in terms of producing a cost-effective, smooth-running service that will meet the needs of the majority, for the majority of the time, a common corporate strategy to promote the type of care that Marie Smith had for all similar clients seems appropriate.

Midwife Phillips had clearly looked after the well-being and the best interests of her patient. So why had Marie Smith complained? It may be that no matter what a professional might do for them some women are never satisfied. Perhaps they ought to realize just what could go wrong and how much their professional midwife had tried to meet all their needs. However, sometimes the midwife's interpretation of her client's needs may not be accurate.

It would be grossly unjust to suggest that the midwife was not acting in what considered to be the best interests of her client. Further, perhaps her own desires for what she felt was good for her patient led her to believe that every patient would want the same and this may not be true. Her own desires for the labour care and outcome may not be exactly the same as those desires of her patient. Before the midwife acts in the best interests of the client she must be sure that the woman is expressing her needs and wants. These 'best interests' need to be clarified and this discussion must include pertinent aspects of maternal and fetal health that the woman may not be in a position to know, as well as the potential conflict that may arise between midwife and medical staff if the midwife were to support the woman, as her advocate, in defiance of medical policy.

The best way to achieve this might be for the woman to put forward her views and wishes and then for the midwife to make available to the woman such information about herself, the events and fetal well-being issues that she may not be in a position to know. Such information given by the midwife must be both factual and without bias. The woman may then express what her best interests, needs and desires are as she sees them. The midwife must then decide, in discussion with the woman, to what extent she feels she can meet her wishes and the degree to which she would act as the woman's advocate should this be put to the test. In this scenario the midwife would be going some way in learning, developing and refining the skills of the art of advocacy.

Constraints on midwifery practice

The UKCC and the profession do not encourage this degree of advocacy from midwives. Both encourage midwives, within the utilitarian organization of the NHS, to maintain the status quo for the good of the majority. The UKCC has much to say about advocacy but it is strangely like a two-way mirror. In the advisory document *Exercising Accountability* (UKCC, 1989) the UKCC's position on advocacy is clearly defined: 'Advocacy is concerned with promoting and safeguarding the well-being and interests of patients and clients.' And goes on to say: 'The practitioner must be sure that it is the interests of the patient or client that are being promoted rather than the patient or client being used as a vehicle for the promotion of personal or sectional professional interests . . .' and reiterates this by adding that advocacy 'is not concerned with conflict for its own sake'. Is the UKCC suggesting here that the midwife would deliberately engage in a potentially employment-threatening exchange for the sheer fun of it? Or, could this be interpreted as advice to the professional not to engage in any battle that might involve conflict with other HCPs? In which case, if an advocate is to be asked not to defend her client's rights, is she an advocate at all? Indeed, the *Exercising Accountability* document does not say the midwife must 'defend', it says be 'concerned with promoting and safeguarding . . .' (UKCC, 1989).

The position is further obscured when the *Code of Professional Conduct* is more closely examined. The practitioner is charged with acting: 'at all times, in such a manner as to: safeguard and promote the interests of individual patients and clients.' Surely these things are intrinsic to the art of advocacy. The document also advises the HCP that advocacy is not a distinct and separate subject but it is an integral and essential aspect of good professional practice. However, the Code also says that the midwife 'shall act, at all times, in such a manner as to: serve the interests of society; justify public trust and confidence, and uphold and enhance the good standing and reputation of the professions' (UKCC, 1992). Defying one practitioner's orders in defence of the request and rights of the patient, even if done in the most gently assertive way, is surely stating clearly that one professional does not agree with another. In the eyes of the patient and the public this situation can hardly appear as both parties being in agreement. The two UKCC recommendations, to be an advocate and uphold the standing of the professions, could, in practice, come into conflict with one another.

Two recent, very public, professional conduct cases serve to demonstrate these ambiguities in practice, those of Graham Pink, working in the care of the elderly, and Jilly Rosser, an independent midwife (see Chapter 12). Both of these cases should encourage midwives to think carefully about the implications of the *Code of Professional Conduct*. But what of the influences of the profession when considering the midwife advocate?

Professional constraints

In the main, midwifery education, midwifery practice and the midwifery ethos of care are steeped in a history of constraints and control. The first Midwives Act of 1902 gave the regulation and control of midwives not to midwives but to medical men and others. The subsequent Acts of Parliament and other pieces of legislation have not seriously sought to redress this position. There is one exception to this; the document *Changing Childbirth* (Department of Health, 1993) stating 10 key targets to be achieved within five years, does seek to make the midwife the lead professional in the care of at least 30% of pregnant women and offers all women more choice, control and continuity in their maternity care. Apart from verbal support and commitment however, there is little concrete assistance from the government. However, this opportunity must be grasped firmly and acted upon by the profession if women are to have more choice and control in their maternity care. This, however, is only one area of midwifery where there are positive developments occurring. With the growth of the NHS, the development of the Trust status system and the movement of midwifery education into larger combined colleges of nursing and midwifery, and soon into higher education, the prospect of midwives being truly self-governing and controlling has never seemed more remote.

Finally, there are other influencing factors on the midwife advocate. These include aspects associated with the ownership of the patient and those of the midwife's working relationships. These are only referred to as they are addressed in Chapter 12.

Birth of the midwife advocate?

Morally many midwives feel they do have a duty to care for their clients and this could be interpreted as a form of moral ownership. Certainly the UKCC encourages this concept in the *Code of Professional Conduct* when it charges each midwife to act at all times to safeguard and promote the interests of their patients and clients, to recognize and respect their uniqueness and dignity and to respond to their needs (UKCC, 1992). Hence, many midwives feel that they are morally and professionally responsible for their clients to the extent that they believe themselves to be, and that they actually are, the woman's advocate.

In an extended research study undertaken to establish midwives' perceptions of the moral rights of pregnant women (Bartter, 1992, unpublished observations), the role of the midwife advocate and the extent to which the midwives would pursue it was examined.

In the study, 214 midwives working in all clinical practice settings in six different institutions returned a completed anonymous questionnaire, which consisted of 45 questions and three comments sections.

The respondent midwives were directly asked: 'As a qualified midwife do you feel you are properly prepared to be the woman's advocate?'; 130 (60·7%) of the 214 midwives responded in the affirmative. Thus, this demonstrated that the majority of midwives say they do feel prepared for their role as midwife advocate. Fifty-one (24%) said no, 22 (10%) were unsure, and 11 (5%) midwives failed to respond to the question.

When the responses were further examined it revealed that midwives with less clinical experience were less sure of this aspect of their role than midwives with more clinical experience.

Other questions that were asked in the study related to midwives defending pregnant women's rights, each with a 'Yes, No, Unsure' tick response.

(1) As a qualified midwife do you feel you are able to defend the rights of the woman to:
    (a) another midwife?
    (b) medical staff?
    (c) midwifery management?
(2) If you think women's rights are being abused, would you voice your concerns outside the profession?
(3) Do you think midwives should be more active in defending the rights of women?
(4) Should the midwife be the professional to defend the rights of women?

(Women in this questionnaire related to pregnant, labouring or postnatal women within the midwife's sphere of practice.)

All these questions attempted to force elaboration and justification by the respondents. In particular, by cross-referencing responses from linked questions, inter-item correlation could be used to establish the reliability of the midwives' responses to questions on their perceived ability to be the woman's advocate and finally to determine to what lengths they would go in pursuing their chosen role of midwife advocate.

Although when directly asked about their stance on advocacy, 130 of the 214 respondents said that they would be the woman's advocate, in questions that relate to them defending the woman's rights to: (a) another midwife, (b) medical staff or (c) to midwifery management, they answered 184, 141 and 144, respectively, that yes, they would defend these rights to their colleagues. This suggests that perhaps they do not realize, or do not include the defence of another's rights as intrinsic to advocacy. When it came to taking the advocacy role to its ultimate conclusion, only 61 (28·5%) midwives said they would voice their concerns about the abuse of their clients' rights outside of the profession. This low percentage indicates a further dimension of the debate on the position and the relationship of midwives in their profession and the UKCC. In addition, of course, it could be seen as further confusion or lack of understanding by midwives about their role as midwife advocate.

A further interesting discovery from this work is that whilst 155 (72·4%) midwives felt that 'yes' the midwife should be more active in ensuring women have rights, only 61 (28·5%) of the midwives felt that they could or would defend these rights outside of the profession. Yet 124 (57·9%) of these very same midwives said that the midwife should be the professional to defend the rights of women and thus to be their advocate.

Clearly, there is an ambiguity here over what the midwives surveyed felt to be the midwife advocate role in principle and what they professed they would actually do in a practical situation. Indeed, only 61 (28·5%) said they would act as a midwife advocate and defend the woman's rights to the absolute point of whistle-blowing in the security of an anonymous questionnaire. One must wonder if this number would be different in reality.

Perhaps what is asked of the midwife is too much, totally unrealistic or even unnecessary. Tschudin (1992) identifies that the position of an advocate is a delicate and fraught one and she says: 'We can only truly be a patient advocate when we are not concerned about our jobs.' In truth, some of the few who have tried to exercise the art of advocacy have found this to be a valid warning. It must also be recognized that the incursion may not just be from the employer or the UKCC, but could be from both.

In addition to this dilemma, Ashton (1992) states that the midwife cannot be the woman's advocate as her professional status, skills and knowledge set her apart from women in general. She goes on to say that the midwife may find that her professional accountability and responsibility make it difficult, if not impossible, for her to support a woman who demands care that is unsafe, or that would lead to the midwife transgressing her Code of Practice. But what if the care was not proven to be unsafe? What if the Codes were likely to be transgressed if she did not respond to her patient's need for care? Would she still be set apart from her client *in general*, and thus be unable to act as advocate? It is conscience easing to put forward the armour of professional status, enhanced skills and greater knowledge as a forced distance.

It could be that midwives are acting paternalistically when they profess that they have a role as client advocate. Thompson (1989) suggests that we may be assuming too much if we counter that every client of the midwife will be in need of an advocate. She says that: 'The mother is not a passive, voiceless "patient". She is usually an adult, self determining, fully conscious person with her own life.... She needs no advocate in the sense of one who speaks for her. She just needs a chance to speak and be heard.' Perhaps then the midwife needs to concentrate more on making time available to listen to her clients. However, just as some women are articulate and autonomous and in control of their childbirth experiences, others are not.

Holmes (1991) argues that the best way to deal with the patient advocate system in the NHS is to have a scheme that is totally separate from the nurse or midwife and independent of the employer and the UKCC's influences on the practitioner. An advocacy system was started in Leeds in 1987, funded by the city council. It works by direct client contact and is solely for the client. The advocate accompanies the client during consultations with doctors, explaining what has been said and putting forward the client's views and wishes. For some people the advocate needs to say nothing, as their presence alone gives clients more confidence to speak for themselves. The advocate also informs clients of their legal and medical rights and maternity advocates are part of the scheme.

Advocacy in midwifery practice, as identified in this work, involves more than this, yet the system is in demand and apparently successful. In addition, although many midwives, in common with nurses, may state that they should be their clients' advocates, it can be argued that sometimes clients need outside support and midwives and nurses are ill trained in this area (Holmes, 1991). How does this help the many maternity units whose clients are not able to use the scheme, or the thousands of midwives who believe that they are, and should be, their client's advocate?

The midwife advocate: a new approach

Perhaps what is needed is a new direction. The legal advocate position and interpretation is not directly transferable into midwifery. We should start again and look at the situation logically and afresh. Midwives clearly need assistance in clarifying their thoughts concerning advocacy in midwifery and midwifery managers need to consider not only their own views, but also the wider implications of a midwife advocate system in practice. An attempt must be made to crystallize the issues by identifying the salient points and the possible constraints and influencing factors involved.

The ideas expressed in *Midwife Advocate New Start Guide* (Bartter, 1994, unpublished observations) could be a starting point in this process. The Guide has two elements to it: both are interrelated and dependent on each other, but each has a slightly different emphasis. The first part is geared toward the individual midwife, the second considers the broader issues, but both elements need to be considered by all, midwives and their managers alike.

Midwives are urged to clarify their personal considerations and think about advocacy in midwifery in general and about their role and responsibilities as a midwife advocate. Those who manage, influence the practice of, or interact with midwives are urged to consider not only their own personal position, but also the wider issues identified and the possible ramifications of promoting, or even discouraging the birth and growth of the midwife advocate concept. Then, each midwife should look deeply into herself and ask herself the following questions:

● What do I feel about advocacy?

- What is my understanding of its implications for me as a midwife?
- What do I consider to be my role and responsibility in this dimension towards my client?
- Do I operate in degrees of advocacy?
- Would I fight the good fight, provided my job is not on the line, or my working relationships under threat?

Although reading and discussion with others may be beneficial and indeed necessary to improve comprehension and clarity, the answer to each of these questions lies deep within the midwife herself. What she must do is to ask, then answer, honestly for herself.

From here she must look at the wider picture and consider the following points.

(1) Does every maternity 'patient' need a midwife advocate?
(2) For those who do, do they need the same service?
(3) What is it that each woman needs?
(4) Is every midwife capable of being or willing to be an advocate?
(5) What are the possible constraints?

- The UKCC and its Codes of Professional behaviour.
- The employee/employer relationship.
- A largely deontological breed of midwife in a mainly utilitarian organization.
- The midwife's working relationships with colleagues and aligned professionals.
- The possible conflict areas between the rights and needs of the mother and the rights and needs of the fetus on physical, moral and philosophical planes.
- The educational and moral stances of the midwife.
- Clarity of perception, so that the midwife knows what the woman wants, and not what she thinks the woman wants.
- Lack of knowledge and research from which to make informed choices.

Conclusion

The points expressed in *Midwife Advocate New Start Guide* (Bartter, 1994, unpublished observations) do not give the answers; they can only direct and nurture growth. The process of growth is not easy.

In this new dawn little is available to help, lead, support and develop each midwife in this uncharted sea. It is unlike anything she has yet been prepared for, but if she reads, learns, reflects and really listens, she will hear what is required of her to fulfil the advocate part of her role. For if the midwife is to strive to be the *midwife advocate—the noble being*, she must take up the challenge of her own volition, fully aware of what is at stake, in the knowledge that although the risks are great, the potential rewards are greater.

References

Ashton, R. (1992). Who Can Speak For Women? *Nursing Times*, **88** (29), p. 70.

Bartter, K. (1994). *Midwife Advocate New Start Guide*. Unpublished.

Bartter, K. (1992). *Moral Rights and Pregnant Women*. M.A. Thesis Unpublished.

Bennett, V. and Brown, L. (1989). *Myles Textbook for Midwives*, 11th edition. Churchill Livingstone.

Currell, R. cited in Alexander, J. *et al*. eds (1990). *Antenatal Care—A Research-Based Approach*. MacMillan Educational Ltd.

Department Of Health. (1993). Changing Childbirth. Report of the Expert Maternity Group. HMSO.

Department of Health. (1994). *The Patient's Charter—Maternity Services*. HMSO.

DuCann, R. (1980). *The Art of The Advocate*. Penguin Books.

Enkin, M., Keirse, M. and Chalmers, I. (1990). *A Guide to Effective Care in Pregnancy and Childbirth*. Oxford University Press.

Garrey, M., Govan, A. D. T., Hodge, C. and Callander, R. (1980). *Obstetrics Illustrated*. 3rd edition. Churchill Livingstone.

Hayward, A. and Sparkes, J. (eds) (1968). *Cassell's English Dictionary*. Cassell.

Henderson, C. (1990). In *Intrapartum Care—A Research-Based Approach*. (J. Alexander *et al*.) MacMillan Educational Ltd.

Holmes, P. (1991). The Patient's Friend. *Nursing Times*, **87** (19), p. 16–17.

House of Commons. (1992). *Winterton Report*. HMSO.

Marshall, M. (1991). Advocacy within the multidisciplinary team. *Nursing Standard*, **6** (10), p. 28–31.

Methven, R. cited in Alexander, J. *et al*. eds (1990). *Antenatal Care—A Research-Based Approach*. MacMillan Educational Ltd.

Silverton, L. (1993). *The Art and Science of Midwifery*. Prentice Hill International (UK) Ltd.

Sleep, J. cited in Alexander, J. *et al*. eds (1990). *Intrapartum Care—A Research-Based Approach*. MacMillan Educational Ltd.

Thompson, A. (1989). Conflict and covenant—ethics in the midwifery curriculum. *Midwives Chronicle & Nursing Notes*, 102 (1217), 191–197.

Tschudin, V. (1992). *Ethics in Nursing*. Heinemann Nursing.

UKCC. (1989). *Exercising Accountability*. UKCC.

UKCC. (1992). *Code of Professional Conduct*. UKCC.

Chapter 14

Ethics in midwifery research

Carolyn Hicks

Introduction

Over the last decade or so increasing pressure has been directed at health care professionals to increase the research base of their practice (e.g. Peckham, 1991; Department of Health, 1993). The reason underpinning these moves stems from the current emphasis on public accountability, in that it is no longer considered acceptable for health care delivery to be founded on ritual and historical precedent but instead should be based on sound empirical evidence. As a result the paramedical professions are being urged to conduct research within their own areas of responsibility in order to challenge existing practices, to identify cost-effective interventions and through these activities to enhance the quality of care. Indeed, so great is the commitment to research that it is stipulated in the International Code of Ethics for Midwives (International Confederation of Midwives, 1993) that midwives should 'develop and share midwifery knowledge through a variety of processes such as peer review and research.' Research and its dissemination are no longer optional niceties but rather the *ethical* responsibility of the midwife.

Acknowledgement of the importance of research-based practice is reflected in the changes to the core curriculum of many midwifery training courses, to incorporate a research skills module. This, together with a shift in health care culture towards evidence-based clinical service, means that many midwives, newly equipped with the necessary skills, are now embarking on research activities at some level. But because midwifery research has as a principal focus of its activities some of the most vulnerable sectors of the population – the fetus, the neonate, the woman in pain or distress – it means that midwives, almost more than many other professional groups, have a particular responsibility to those who are participants in the research. Therefore, the midwife-researcher must recognize these responsibilities by ensuring that she is fully aware of the ethical principles which must, of necessity, guide the research. This chapter is an attempt to bring together the most important of these considerations as they apply to midwifery research.

Ethical issues in research

The overriding concern of any researcher using human subjects must be the protection of their rights, dignity and physical and psychological welfare. Any activity that compromises the participants in any of these ways must be regarded as ethically suspect. Consequently, ethical dilemmas have the capacity to impinge upon every stage of the research project. It is therefore imperative that both the reader of midwifery research and the researcher herself are aware of where these dilemmas might influence the essential decision making. Asking the following questions of the research may act as a useful aid:

- what is the research topic?
- who is to conduct the research?
- who will benefit from the research?
- where will the research be conducted?
- how will the participants be treated?
- how will the research be carried out?
- how will the findings be disseminated?

The ethical considerations inherent to every question will be considered separately.

What is the research topic?

Research is about asking questions and finding answers to those questions in a systematic and objective way. However, the sort of research question that is being asked may raise at the outset a number of ethical issues, which may have to be balanced against the anticipated benefits of the research.

Any research should start out with the implicit assumption that it will have some value to someone. Research for its own sake is unlikely to be sanctioned by ethical committees, especially where human participation is involved; for example, any proposed midwifery intervention which had no theoretical or experiential support to attest to its potential usefulness might well be rejected. Allied to this is the issue of resources, which should not be wasted on pointless exercises unlikely to contribute to the corpus of midwifery knowledge.

Many research topics are inherently controversial and potentially very damaging. Investigations into racial differences inevitably arouse objections, in part because the findings can be misrepresented as a means of introducing discriminatory and abusive practices. Research which probes into embarrassing or intimate aspects of a participant's experiences is also highly questionable, since it will almost certainly cause distress and anxiety. Midwifery research may frequently be involved with private aspects of an individual's behaviour and lifestyle, such as sexual behaviour, drug abuse, AIDS, and so on. This is not to suggest that research concerning these topics should be abandoned, but rather that a careful cost–benefit analysis should be the first stage, so that the potential advantages of the research can be weighed against the disadvantages to the participants. If the midwife-researcher decides that the pros outweigh the cons, then the research methodology selected must reflect the sensitive nature of the research question using only those procedures that will minimize participant distress.

Who is to conduct the research?

Good research is only possible if there is mutual respect and confidence between the researcher and the participant. Therefore, anybody who conducts research, especially that which involves human subjects, must be skilled, competent and able to do so. This means that the midwife-researcher should take responsibility for ensuring that her understanding of research procedures in the very widest sense is as full and comprehensive as possible. Where the responsibility for the research is shared, then any midwife who observes a co-researcher acting incompetently or engaging in malpractice, which is in contravention of accepted ethical conduct, must be prepared to take appropriate action. This in itself poses potential difficulties, particularly if the offending co-worker is senior to the midwife. However, the overriding consideration must always be the welfare of the research participants and anything that threatens this must be curtailed. Failure or refusal to accept responsibility for co-workers must consequently be construed as a potential ethical problem.

Related to this is the issue of sponsored research. Science is supposed to be objective and independent by its very nature, but this position may be undermined if the research is financed by an organization or company which has a vested interest in the outcome. Where the researcher is in the paid employ of such a company, their objectivity as a researcher may be influenced by their dependency on the company for a job. This is not to suggest dishonesty but merely that the freedom of the researcher to report and publish *all* the salient findings might be limited by the company's need to present its product to potential customers in the most seductive and enticing light. It is indeed well-known within medical circles that there have been many instances in the past where adverse results have been suppressed in order to safeguard the product under investigation. Such control over the research and the motivations underlying the control constitute a very serious ethical problem for many researchers, particularly in times when alternative employment may be hard to find. Therefore, the role and position of the researcher is a critical one. In an ideal world, the researcher is competent, autonomous and independent. In reality, she may be, 'the "hired hand" doing the bidding of the paymaster … or … simply ammunition wagons, loaded with powerful knowledge just waiting to be used, whether the users are the "good guys" or the "bad guys".' (Robson, 1993).

It should always be remembered, too, that the investigator holds special powers. The researcher is in a position of influence and authority over the participants, and this position is exaggerated in medically related research when a clear dominant–subordinate relationship normally and inevitably exists between the health care professional and the patient. In these circumstances, the patient/client may feel under obligation to the researcher and so may comply with research demands simply to ensure that they will not be disadvantaged in other aspects of their care. This places enormous responsibilities on the researcher to ensure that she does not abuse her position of authority either to coerce patients to participate or to influence the participants' responses in a way that benefits the research. If the researcher cannot guarantee that these malpractices will not occur, then it is essential that a disinterested colleague who is not directly responsible for the research or patient's care conducts the study. Under these conditions it is easier for the patient/client to withdraw from the study.

Who will benefit from the research?

The question of who will benefit from the research may well give rise to grandiose, if somewhat naive, answers of 'humanity' and 'medical science'. More realistically, it is likely that only a small subgroup of the population will derive any short- or long-term good; for example, if the midwife-researcher is interested in looking at the impact of a specially prepared exercise regimen on the presentation of a breech baby, then the results are only likely to advantage other pregnant women with breech presentation fetuses. This does not invalidate the research by any means, but it is important that the beneficiaries of the study are honestly identified. The reason for this relates back to the point about who conducts the research. If the investigator is in the paid employ of a large corporation, for instance an infant food manufacturer, then it is quite conceivable that the principal beneficiary may be the sponsor, especially if restrictions are imposed regarding the nature, conduct and publication of the research. Another beneficiary may be the researcher who, if she provides her employer with the desired results, may get an extension to her contract. The implicit cynicism in this message is becoming an increasing reality now that the public service relies more and more heavily on private companies rather than on government departments for its research money.

Even if the midwife is an independent and autonomous researcher with obligations to no one and nothing but the scientific truth, it is still conceivable that the benefits accruing from the research will be greater for the investigator than for the investigated. Research carries considerable kudos in most professional domains and consequently any researcher who generates a set of interesting results may gain in prestige, peer opinion and even career prospects.

The message in this cynical tale is simply that any potential benefits that might accrue to the investigator, the sponsor, or even to the knowledge base of midwifery must be very carefully and honestly balanced against the nature and conduct of the project and its impact on the participants.

Where will the research be conducted?

Working on the assumption that midwifery research has the potential to improve client well-being and care, the question of where to conduct the research must, of necessity, raise key ethical considerations, since participating venues may automatically have a potential advantage over those units not selected for study.

Conversely, the selection of a particular venue for the research may fuel an already explosive situation, simply by its focus of attention; for example, a hypothetical study conducted in a large urban psychiatric unit which found that post-partum psychosis was significantly more prevalent in a particular ethnic group might inflame racial tension and discrimination. Alternatively, targeting particular geographical areas for health education literature on smoking and alcohol abuse during pregnancy might inadvertently suggest that some social classes are more likely to abuse the fetus in these ways. Once again, whatever the potential for difficulty, it must be weighed against the wider value of the information that can be gained from the project.

There is one further point regarding the selection of a research venue. Many units are more than happy to co-operate with research activities simply because there will be tangible gains for them, at least in the short term. One example of this might be the (temporary) provision of an ultrasound scanner in a remote rural health centre, in order to look at its impact on early identification of fetal abnormality in a population too distant from the main hospital to take advantage of its services. For the duration of the project, the centre, at no cost to itself, would have additional screening resources. This can of course be construed as a necessary, and useful to the unit, aspect of the research. To those of a more cynical disposition, it could be seen as a bribe to participate. Even if no technical equipment goes with participation, it is quite likely that the researcher might constitute an extra pair of hands or other resource. Are these just part of the deal or does it smack of the sort of coercion used to encourage prisoners to take part in dangerous drug trials in exchange for privileges? Clearly, then, the wider implications of a research project must be considered fully.

How will the participants be treated?

The research participants (often called subjects) are the cornerstone of any study and the protection of their rights, dignity and well-being must be the primary concern of the researcher. Indeed, the major responsibility of any ethical committee is to ensure that the subjects are treated in a way that does not compromise any aspect of their mental and physical welfare. Treatment of the participants is heavily bound up with the type of methodology adopted in the study and this is dealt with in the next section. However, there are issues that will be discussed under this heading.

The main focus of the World Medical Association's Declaration of Helsinki (1975) is the treatment of the research participants; who will and will not be included, the privacy of their behaviour and their general well-being. Similarly, both the British Psychological Society's (1985) and the American Psychological Association's (1987) agreed guidelines for research have a principal concern for the welfare of the subjects and any intending midwife researcher should study these documents in detail. In midwifery research, these concerns are heightened because of the vulnerability of the likely research participants. The particular ethical problems associated with midwifery research relate to the issue of *informed consent*, which requires that the participants knowingly, freely and rationally agree to take part in the research. Obviously, in the case of a baby, embryo or fetus, it is the parents who are asked for their agreement, and while this is the logical and proper alternative, it does nonetheless raise special concerns amongst ethical committees and researchers.

The point about informed consent is a fundamental one for ethically acceptable research. Every risk involved in the research must be properly explained and understood. In addition, the procedures involved must be described fully where possible, but this in itself may provoke debate. Many studies, for example, would be rendered valueless if the intentions and methods were outlined to subjects beforehand, simply because advance knowledge may create a set of expectations in the participants which may distort the outcome. To illustrate this point, a study with clinical midwives (Hicks, 1992) investigated how the sample viewed research conducted by midwives as opposed to that carried out by doctors. Two articles on the same midwifery topic were distributed to the group. However, half the group were told that the first article had been conducted by a midwife and the second by a doctor, while for the rest of the group, the information was reversed. The midwives were asked to read both articles and then to evaluate them according to a number of specified criteria. The evaluations of the articles allegedly conducted by the midwife were significantly lower on a number of key criteria than were those of the articles purported to have been carried out by the doctor. The methodology here could legitimately be criticized for its duplicity, since the sample was deceived regarding the authorship of the papers. However, it is self-evident that had the group been informed of the true authorship in advance of the study, then the research would have lost its whole point. Many other examples abound where the methodology involves deceiving the participants in some way as a necessary expedient of a valid research design. Studies that involve placebos, for example, are good illustrations of necessary duplicity. Inevitably, if subjects were told in advance that the treatment they were receiving was worthless, it would be unlikely that there would be any perceptible impact of the placebo condition.

While deception may be an unavoidable aspect of the methodology it is not necessarily desirable, since tricking innocent participants in this way cannot conceivably be regarded as ideal and may have serious long-term psychological and physical implications for the participants (see Bakhurst, 1992 and Jackson, 1993 for a debate of this issue). However, as Coolican (1992) implies, there may be no methodologically acceptable alternative. The resolution of this problem again revolves around a full cost–benefit analysis; do the anticipated benefits of the study outweigh the disadvantages of the design?

Whatever the level of deception, however, it is imperative that the researcher debriefs the subjects at the conclusion of the project. The debriefing must reveal the real purpose and aims of the project and, very importantly, must ensure that the subjects feel the same about themselves when they leave as they did when they arrived. However, this in itself may involve further deception. A hypothetical example concerning pain relief in labour might involve the comparison of a placebo with a true analgesic on reported pain levels. The debriefing would reveal the true nature of the study and some feedback to individual women about their pain responses. Would it be acceptable to tell someone that they made 'more fuss', or screamed louder or complained more vociferously than anyone else in the study? The point here is that to preserve an individual's dignity there may be some circumstances that require the investigator to modify the feedback. Where the midwife researcher is uncertain about the nature and extent of any duplicitous procedures used, then advice should be sought from experienced and impartial colleagues who have no investment in the study's outcomes. The role of the ethical committee is also important in these circumstances, where the central guiding principle is always the minimization of any potential short-, medium- or long-term mental and physical distress for the subjects.

In paramedical research, there are also the possible problems surrounding the use of new treatments, the side-effects of which are unknown, of denying someone a treatment that has demonstrable value or of using overly intrusive techniques. While these issues are fundamentally methodological in nature, they do have implications for participant welfare. Lest the reader should protest that such issues are well outside the province of midwifery research, some illustrations may be useful. As an illustration of the first point, take a project whose focus is the use of a specially designed exercise programme intended to invert known breech presentations to cephalic presentations. It seems innocuous enough but the procedure would involve selecting a group of women and asking them to comply with an exercise regimen assumed (at least theoretically) to be useful, but without any evidence as to its value. *Could* it lead to adverse side-effects? With regard to the second point, withholding treatment is a standard practice in any study that involves the use of a control group; for example, if the midwife was interested in assessing the benefits of counselling for women who have delivered handicapped babies, it would be necessary to look at comparable women who received no such support. Is it ethical to withhold this intervention? This issue is discussed more fully in the next section. The third point regarding the use of overly intrusive techniques can be illustrated by the use of questionnaires which investigate the respondent's previous or current sexual activities, substance abuse, and so on. Each of these examples illustrates the particular problems that paramedical research faces when attempting to find a compromise position between ethical and scientific acceptability.

Sometimes the research methodology involves the observation of participants in naturalistic settings. However, if subjects are aware that they are being watched, it is highly likely that their behaviour will change significantly, thereby undermining the naturalistic nature of the study. Consequently, participants may be observed without being aware of it. This may be considered an invasion of privacy, even when the behaviour seems innocent, but it is undoubtedly unacceptable if private and personal behaviours are under scrutiny. Consider, for example, a study which looks at the responses of a woman and her partner to a male midwife who assists during the second stage of labour. It is conceivable that the investigator might record a number of verbal and non-verbal responses in the couple when a shift change results in the arrival of a male midwife. The situation might be observed via a one-way mirror (a very typical way of conducting an observational study), which would enable the investigator to conduct the study without being seen and therefore without any of the participants being aware of what was going on. Such an 'intrusion' into a very private and personal event without prior permission is a serious contravention of ethical codes of conduct. And yet, the available evidence suggests that not only is it essential that naturalistic events are recorded without participants' knowledge, since awareness will distort the behaviour, but also because there again appears to be no satisfactory methodological alternative (Coolican, 1992). As with other dilemmas arising out of the conflict between sound methodology and ethical acceptability, it is important that any studies involving non-voluntary participation are discussed with colleagues who are experienced in research matters. Generally, however, the British Psychological Society's Ethical Guidelines suggest that observational research is only acceptable in those situations when the participants would *expect* to be observed by strangers, and also that due consideration should be taken with respect to cultural and local mores and values since it is easy to infringe these quite unwittingly.

It should be pointed out here that if any research procedure is likely to cause distress of any sort, then it is essential that only the minimum number of participants are used. This clearly flies in the face of common folklore, which assumes that the greater the number of subjects the better the study. This is a mythology which is neither valid from a methodological viewpoint nor acceptable from an ethical one. While it is clear that there must be a mid-position between sound research procedures and ethical considerations, the potential impact on the participants must always be a primary concern.

Where some discomfort is inevitable, the researcher must recognize the right of the subjects to refuse to participate. In order to exercise that right though, the subjects must be fully informed about the risks and their right to withdraw from the research at any point and for whatever reason. There may also be situations when the investigator decides to terminate the study, because the observed problems are greater than anticipated.

Particular difficulties arise when subjects are paid or remunerated in some way for their participation (e.g. Harries and Edwards, 1994). This situation can create an employer/employee relationship with an implicit contractual obligation. In these instances, the 'employer' may feel empowered to make excessive or unreasonable demands of the 'employee', who, in turn, may feel obliged to tolerate unacceptable procedures or produce the responses desired by the 'employer' but which may not be their honest reactions.

The need to protect the privacy and confidentiality of subjects is a key issue in all research. All participants have the right to anonymity, privacy and confidentiality and if this cannot be guaranteed, then the subject must be informed immediately and given the right to withdraw from the project. Any participant who has been deceived about this point has the right to witness the destruction of any data and information concerning them. There may also be a case for litigation. However, sometimes the investigator may wish to follow up individual cases, which is impossible if anonymity is absolute. In these cases, the researcher may eliminate any identification of the individual by name, but instead may use numerical or alphabetic code. In this way the privacy of the individual is maintained while allowing for possible follow-up.

The issue of confidentiality, while a crucial one, has its own conflicts. If a participant has performed particularly well, honourably or diligently during a project, is it not reasonable that she should be rewarded? For example, an anonymous survey of working practices among community midwives might reveal a small cohort who routinely operate over and above the call of duty, not only in terms of the hours worked, but also in the tasks undertaken and the results obtained. It is a cogent argument that they should have just reward, but this is clearly impossible if the study conforms to the confidentiality rule. Conversely, if the survey found that a small number of community midwives were behaving negligently or improperly, then the protection of their identity also serves to perpetuate their malpractice. Sometimes a moral dilemma emerges. Supposing a researcher found that a midwife or client had undisclosed AIDS, and that they were putting at risk many of those with whom they came into close contact. How is confidentiality to be treated where there is a substantial threat to human life?

During research, particularly that in the health care arena, it is quite likely that the researcher may come across a problem of which the participant is unaware. In such circumstances, it is the responsibility of the researcher to inform the subject of this problem if it is believed that by withholding this information the subject's well-being may be jeopardized. Sometimes as a result of these problems being disclosed the participant seeks the advice of the researcher. Only if the researcher is fully qualified should this advice be proffered, otherwise the appropriate professional help should be sought.

How will the research be carried out?

Research involves the midwife asking questions about her practice or observations and then using scientific methods to answer those questions. There are two basic research methodologies available to the midwife-researcher, each of which stems from a different set of assumptions. These methodologies are called *qualitative* and *quantitative* methods. The former involves the naturalistic study of the client/patient as a whole person (as opposed to a set of behaviours or symptoms) within a social framework. In this way, the researcher attempts to gain insight into the client/patient's subjective thoughts, feelings and experiences within a given set of circumstances; for example, the midwife-researcher might want to explore the birth experiences of a group of elderly primigravid women and so might interview them within six hours of delivery to record their emotional, psychological and attitudinal responses to the birth. To conduct this research, the midwife-researcher would, of necessity, be in close personal interaction with the mothers, she would record their descriptions of their reactions to the birth, and from these descriptions she would interpret the group's responses in order to provide insights into the highly personal and subjective experience of giving birth. The researcher's interpretations would be discussed with the mothers to see whether they made any sense or had any meaning for them. The more the researcher and the mothers agree with regard to their interpretation of the birth experience, the more likely it is that the interpretations are valid and accurate. The value of this study would be primarily in the enhanced understanding of what the birth experience means for elderly primigravid women, so that health care delivery in this context can be modified to improve the client's experiences. Such an approach to midwifery research is very commonly used; for example, Lydon-Rochelle and Albers (1993) found in a survey conducted over five years that 67% of midwifery research used a descriptive approach to research. One reason for this is the evident value it has within midwifery practice, where the closeness of the relationship between the client and the midwife is an essential part of the delivery of care.

Another reason for the popularity of this approach relates to the fact that it is, by definition, normalistic. This means that there is no manipulation of treatment procedures, no intervention in the service delivery and no withholding therapy or care. Consequently, there may well be fewer ethical problems arising out of the conduct of the research programme. However, any study that focuses on the most intimate thoughts and experiences of an individual must have a fundamental regard for their privacy and well-being. The very content of the interview or questionnaire might be distressing and therefore the participants must always be aware of their right not to participate without fear that their refusal might compromise their care. Moreover, the close relationship that qualitative research requires between the participant and researcher means that objective interpretation of events might be very difficult to achieve. In consequence, bias might creep into the conclusions, with possible deleterious impact on subsequent health care. To illustrate this, take a hypothetical example of a research study into the quality of antenatal care for lesbian mothers. The midwife-researcher might be motivated to conduct this because of the adverse antenatal experiences of a close personal friend who is lesbian. With the best will in the world, it would be difficult for the midwife-researcher to start the project on neutral territory, and so her potential for misinterpreting events as a result of her attitudes, beliefs and expectations must of necessity be fairly high. This is not to suggest that the researcher would enter the research intending to distort the evidence, but rather that the human element which adds richness to the qualitative approach may also detract from the objectivity of the recordings. Thus, in this study, when the researcher interviews a lesbian mother, any statement or viewpoint the subject proffers which accords with what the researcher expects or hopes to hear may be overemphasized in the report. Conversely, any disclosure which disagrees with the researcher's expectations may be underreported. Consequently, the findings from the study may be a distortion of reality and may, therefore, misinform future health-care planning with regard to antenatal provision. Improvements in objectivity might be achieved by having additional researchers present, so that some counterbalancing of bias and view can be achieved, or alternatively a totally independent, unconnected researcher who has no vested interest in the outcome of the study could be used.

Other methodological problems are associated with qualitative research. The impact of an observer on the subjects' behaviour, for example, has already been discussed. In addition, there are difficulties associated with attempting to procure returns in questionnaire surveys. Quite often the initial number of returns is too low to be of any value and so the researcher sends out reminders to the non-returners. But should they be harassed in this way? Many people feel intimidated by this sort of pressure and while good return rate may be highly desirable from the researcher's perspective, the individual cost to the recipients of written or telephone reminders might be unacceptably high, particularly if the recipient is already vulnerable.

The second major methodological approach is the *quantitative method*, which as its name suggests involves the collection and analysis of numerical data. Such a technique is often anathema to the health care professions whose tradition has been founded on quality and intuition, rather than on formal quantification. This approach has its roots firmly fixed in science. It involves the objective, detached measurement of events as a means of testing hypotheses. To do this, the researcher has to control the research situation, and manipulate the procedures in order that cause and effect relationships can be identified. Any findings emerging from the study can be used to predict and control future health care delivery. Just reading this synopsis of the scientific method arouses immediate ethical queries. The vocabulary alone ('control', 'manipulate') is indicative that research participants have lost their freedom to choose and this may be a serious contravention of proper ethical codes of conduct. Whether such an approach can ever be justified in midwifery may be the target of legitimate debate.

However, the value of this approach in adding to the knowledge base of midwifery is beyond dispute. Questions arise such as:

- which care approach is best for a given group of clients?
- which people are most likely to benefit from a particular intervention?
- what is the most likely course of a specified problem?
- which interventions are most cost-effective?

These can be answered by the scientific method and are of vital importance if midwifery care is to be systematized and improved. However, the scientific method involved in answering them may raise ethical problems whose gravity may offset any benefits. The use of a hypothetical example may be the best illustration of this point.

A midwife working in the antenatal clinic of a large teaching hospital is interested in looking at the psychological impact of chorionic villus sampling (CVS) on maternal well-being. Her hypothesis is that CVS has a beneficial effect on maternal psychological state. She decides to select a group of women who have opted for CVS and to assess their psychological state before and after CVS, thus.

A group of women has:

Pre-CVS   Post-CVS
measure of   →   CVS   → measure of
psychological state   psychological state.

By comparing the before and after measures of psychological state, the midwife believes that she will be able to determine the impact of CVS. However, a colleague points out that psychological state might have altered anyway, simply as a function of the stage of the pregnancy. Since CVS is typically performed at a point when the woman has adjusted to the knowledge of being pregnant it is quite likely that psychological state would start to improve at around this time and that any changes observed in the group may reflect this rather than the impact of CVS. To get round this, the midwife-researcher decides to study another group of women at the same stage of pregnancy but who do not undergo CVS, the control group. The research design now looks like this.

Group 1

Pre-CVS			Post-CVS
measure of	→	CVS	→ measure of
psychological state			psychological state.

Group 2 (control)

First			Second
measure of	→	No CVS	→ measure of
psychological state			psychological state.

If the two groups of women are the same in all respects bar the CVS, then any differences between them at second testing must be the result of the CVS. By using this improved design, the researcher can indeed answer the question regarding the positive impact CVS has on the woman's psychological state. However, the devil's advocate colleague then points out that the group of women who were offered CVS had all belonged to an 'at-risk' category of mothers who had received genetic counselling prior to pregnancy. The group who did not receive CVS had not been drawn from this category and therefore the study was not comparing like with like. The midwife-researcher reconsiders the design and decides to select a second group of women from the at-risk register, but to withhold the option of CVS. This design now compares like with like but also has some very grave ethical problems. Is it acceptable to withhold treatment, intervention or screening from anyone? This problem is a very difficult one indeed and is a characteristic of any study that uses a control (or no treatment) group in this way. In such cases, a number of expedients can be adopted. One typical option would be a comparison of *two* interventions rather than a comparison of *one* intervention with a *control* or *no intervention* group. In this example, then, the impact of CVS would be compared with another similar screening procedure (i.e. amniocentesis) to see if one approach was more beneficial psychologically than the other. However, this option is not particularly useful in this study, since amniocentesis is carried out at a later stage in pregnancy and therefore once again, like is not being compared with like. Nonetheless, the use of a second treatment group for the purposes of comparison can be a valuable and ethically more acceptable option than a control group in many studies and should always be considered where the use of a no-treatment group is dubious.

Another alternative to the predicament of the control group would be to use women in the 'at risk' group, who had voluntarily decided *not* to have CVS. This is a naturalistic choice which does not force women into situations against their wishes. The revised design now uses two groups of women, both at risk from genetic problems and both at a similar stage of pregnancy. However, one group has elected to have CVS and the other has not. How acceptable is this design now? The devil's advocate could legitimately continue to criticize. The group who chooses CVS, she points out, are likely to do so because they *expect* that the procedure will have some benefit to them psychologically, by providing the knowledge either that the fetus is normal or that there is a problem about which a decision must be made. Either way, the group believes knowledge to be a useful and beneficial outcome to the screening. Therefore, in the group that has CVS there is an expectation of benefit which may not be present in the control group, and it is this expectation rather than the actual procedure or its outcome that has the effect. In order to overcome the problem of expectation in a study, *placebo* groups are often used. This procedure involves giving some subjects an entirely worthless intervention to establish whether the participants' expectation of benefit actually produces any change. This precaution is commonly used in drug trials. If a new drug is being tested, patients taking the drug may show an improvement *simply* because they expect any treatment to benefit them. In order to counteract this problem, some subjects are given useless saline injections, or sugar pills to see if they have an effect. The success of the placebo rests upon the patients' ignorance of what it is they are taking, and therefore, there is an element of deception in the procedure which may have ethical implications.

If this design is incorporated into the present study then a further group of women would have unwittingly to experience a fake vaginal investigation using instruments and procedures comparable to those used during actual CVS. The study now looks like this:

Group 1

Pre-CVS			Post-CVS
assessment of	→	true CVS →	assessment of
psychological state			psychological state.

Group 2

Pre-test			Post-test
assessment of	→	fake CVS	→ assessment of
psychological state			psychological state.

Group 3 (control)

First			Second test
test of	→	no CVS	→ assessment of
psychological state			psychological state.

Methodologically, the study has been substantially improved, but these improvements have introduced some very serious ethical concerns. Because neither fake nor true CVS procedures can be forced on the women who have decided to have no screening at all (Group 3), to introduce a placebo procedure means that a selection of women who believed they were choosing CVS will unknowingly have to undergo a useless or even risky procedure. This not only raises the debate discussed earlier regarding deception of participants but also puts physical and psychological welfare at risk through the application of a useless investigation. Moreover, how would the researcher decide who should undergo the true CVS and who the fake? Conventional research procedures would suggest that the women are randomly selected for either condition and in this way they would all have an equal chance of receiving the true CVS. However, it is questionable ethically whether anyone who desires a statutory treatment or intervention should be excluded from having it. Individual access to appropriate treatment must form a central aspect of any debate regarding research methodology involving randomized trials.

Within this example runs the suggestion that perfect research methodology can only be achieved at the expense of ethical considerations and vice versa. However, real-world research in whatever domain must effect an acceptable balance between the validity of the research procedures and adherence to ethical guidelines. Midwifery research, like all other research whose focus is applied, must select a compromise position which recognizes the mutual limitations that ethics and methodology impose on each other.

There are, of course, other techniques of research such as correlational designs and single case studies which all have their pitfalls. While problems outlined in this section also apply to these designs, the reader might like to look at Polgar and Thomas (1992) for a more detailed discussion of their particular characteristics.

How will the findings be disseminated?

If research is to inform and improve midwifery practice, then it must be properly and widely disseminated in order that other practitioners can evaluate the findings and incorporate them appropriately into their own service delivery. Thus there is a moral obligation on both the researchers to report and the practitioners to evaluate. However, this can only be done if the research is fairly and properly recorded.

The current pressure on researchers in all areas to publish research means that there is a potential for bias and corruption. To comply with central government pressure for an increase in research output, it is conceivable that three types of problem might emerge.

(1) Researchers might report incomplete research before the findings have been thoroughly verified.
(2) They might break up the data set in order to increase the number of papers and in so doing might present a set of results which are distorted, clinically meaningless or not representative of the whole picture.
(3) Researchers might fabricate data or 'massage' results.

Therefore, researchers have a responsibility to ensure that what is published is a full and fair account of the outcome of their research. The results should be interpreted as objectively as possible and the conclusions should not be extravagant. These points become difficult if a project has been sponsored by a government department or commercial organization which has an investment in the outcome. In such cases it has been known for contradictory or unacceptable findings to be suppressed, in order to protect the agency.

It is therefore important that the researcher retains the right to report accurately the results of sponsored work as long as the findings do not *unnecessarily* compromise the sponsor. As with all other aspects of research, confidentiality should not be breached in the report, and the identity of all participants should be protected unless they have given their written consent to the contrary.

As with all written work, plagiarism is absolutely unacceptable. If quotations or excerpts are to be used, appropriate authorization and proper protocol should be observed. And, of course, the researcher should always be prepared to allow access to the raw data. Cravenness in this regard breeds suspicion, not only about the researcher's integrity, but also about both method and findings.

Conclusions

Any research using human subjects carries obligations to protect their rights, dignity and welfare. Midwifery, with its involvement with vulnerable client groups, has a particular responsibility to follow appropriate ethical guidelines in order to safeguard the participants. This chapter has outlined where the major ethical obstacles arise in midwifery research. It must be emphasized that there are no definitive rules regarding ethical dilemmas and their solutions. Each problem requires negotiation, careful consideration and compromise. In consequence, then, the following points must be regarded as basic guidelines for conducting ethically acceptable research.

(1) Always obtain full and informed consent from participants; try never to deceive or coerce them in any way.
(2) Always keep the dignity and welfare of the subjects paramount; never diminish, embarrass or compromise them.
(3) Always protect the participants' confidentiality and privacy.
(4) Ensure that the participants know that they can withdraw from the research at any time without sanction.
(5) Always consult with relevant authorities and committees to obtain the necessary approval before embarking on research.
(6) Always discuss with experienced independent others any methodological issues that might compromise the participants.
(7) Be as fair, accurate and objective as possible.

Openness, honesty and integrity breed trust and respect between professionals and client groups. Any profession wishing to pursue research must recognize that the privilege of research is earned through scrupulous behaviour and carries with it both ethical and moral obligations.

References

American Psychological Association. (1987). *Casebook on Ethical Principles of Psychologists*. American Psychological Association.
Bakhurst, D. (1992). On lying and deceiving. *J. Med. Ethics*, **18**, 63–66.
British Psychological Society. (1985). A code of conduct for psychologists. *Bull. Br. Psychol. Soc.*, **38**, 41–43.
Coolican, H. (1992). *Research Methods and Statistics in Psychology*. Hodder and Stoughton.

Department of Health. (1993). *Report of the Task force on the Strategy for Research in Nursing Midwifery and Health Visiting*, Department of Health.

Harries, U. and Edwards, J. (1994). Gift or gain. *Health Service Journal*, 26–27.

Hicks, C. M. (1992). Research in midwifery: Are midwives their own worst enemies? *Midwifery*, 8, 12–18.

International Confederation of Midwives. (1993). *International Code of Ethics for Midwives*. I.C.M.

Jackson, J. (1993). On the morality of deception—does method matter? A reply to David Bakhurst. *J. Med. Ethics*, 19, 183–187.

Lydon-Rochelle, M. and Albers, L. (1993). Research trends in the Journal of Nurse-Midwifery 1987–1992. *J. Nurse-Midwifery*, 38 (6), 343–348.

Peckham, M. (1991). *Research for Health: a Research and Development Strategy for the NHS*. HMSO.

Polgar, S. and Thomas, S. A. (1992). *Introduction to Research in the Health Sciences*. Churchill-Livingstone.

Robson, C. (1993). *Real World Research*. Blackwell.

World Medical Association. (1975). *Declaration of Helsinki*. Royal Medical Association.

Chapter 15

Researching sensitive issues

Hazel McHaffie

Introduction

Throughout their training, midwives are taught to identify a problem and attempt to solve it. Researchers, on the other hand, are encouraged to stand back and observe and note what is taking place but not to 'interfere' lest they influence the dynamics of any situation and jeopardize the integrity of their study. But researchers as well as clinicians are sometimes privy to confidences and information which may have a profound effect on them, and serious consequences for other people.

For researchers investigating areas where potentially damaging information is divulged, a real dilemma may present. How far should they go in preserving confidences? When does their duty as a human being supersede their professional obligations to their respondents? At what point does the danger to life or well-being take precedence over the quality of the data produced? How far should they allow their own values, beliefs and interests to be compromised?

To some extent almost all research with human beings involves asking oneself just where the balance lies. Questions concern harm and benefit; privacy and confidentiality; informed consent and deception, and social control (Kelman, 1982). There are social and moral obligations that relate both to the personal relationships a researcher develops with people in the field, and to the purpose and conduct of the study; for example, how much does a researcher disclose of his or her own agenda and experience? Does sharing personal detail bias respondents or facilitate an honest exchange?

Encouraging respondents to gain insight into their feelings, or to relive painful experiences may provide rich data but what happens to the respondent after the interview? How far does the interviewer's responsibility stretch in the therapeutic direction, especially if he or she has had no training in such matters?

In enquiries about sensitive topics, the questions can become deeply searching. The usual basic and underlying issues are highlighted with particular clarity when seen against the backcloth of threat or secrecy. From the participants' point of view, there may be a risk of powerful emotions being generated or exposed, of loss of respect, and of shame, guilt or public exposure. For the researcher, taboos and restrictions may limit openness. As a consequence, researchers may sanitize their reports. Funding agencies may issue embargoes to suppress sensitive or potentially threatening findings. Gatekeepers may require the investigators to hide or disguise facts to accommodate the host institution's own agenda. Straightforward courtesy and sensitivity may dictate that a veil be drawn over parts of the research simply to protect the finer feelings of other human beings. If a subject is also topical, there is the additional risk of discomforting distortion by the media. Accordingly, much may be left unsaid.

Indeed, much *has* been left unsaid in the course of research carried out in sensitive areas over the years. Furthermore, serious academic attempts to 'tell it like it really is' have on occasions been thwarted because of the 'concealed micropolitics of research' (Punch, 1986). Colleagues, editors and publishers have fought shy of contentious material. As a result, student researchers and others have not always benefited as they might from the wisdom gained in the fierce fire of actual experience. This chapter attempts to address some of the issues raised by research of this nature.

Sensitive topics and the degree of threat

Sensitive areas for research include both topics that touch deep-seated emotions, and those that involve behaviours which are intimate, incriminating or possibly discreditable. Although all research may imply some cost to those participating, in sensitive areas the price is recognized as particularly high. A substantial degree of threat exists for those being studied. And there is a burden to be carried by the investigator too.

Such research may raise methodological problems as well as ethical or legal ones, and the difficulties may occur at almost any stage of the research process. That is not to say that such research should not be undertaken, although some researchers have suggested that certain areas should not be subjected to close scrutiny (MacIntyre, 1982):

> The study of taboos by anthropologists and of privacy by sociologists show how important it is for a culture that certain areas of personal and social life should be specially protected. Intimacy cannot exist where everything is disclosed, sanctuary cannot be sought where no place is inviolate, integrity cannot be seen to be maintained—and therefore cannot in certain cases be maintained—without protection from illegitimate pressures.

However, a cogent argument can be put forward for research into people's private lives. It can be justified, not only on the basis that it will substantially increase knowledge, but also on the grounds that the process itself may indeed have effects of great benefit to the respondents themselves. In my own work amongst mothers with very low birth weight babies, the women frequently commented on the therapeutic effect of sharing their anxieties, anger and frustration. Some indeed volunteered that talking through these issues with me helped them to keep tensions with their partners in check and to avoid actually harming the baby. Sometimes catharsis is more desirable than sanctuary (Lee and Renzetti, 1993). The skill lies in achieving a healthy balance between maximum validity and benefit, and minimum harm.

In conventional positivist theory: 'The investigator's task is to discover that which is hidden or kept secret by subjects (or that which remains unknown to them) and to hold these discovered truths, these facts, to the light of scientific scrutiny. Secrecy has no permanent place in this form of scientific enterprise' (Mitchell, 1991). But a moment's sober reflection will reveal that secrecy pervades human relations and it would be arrogant to believe that a researcher either could or should uncover all that a respondent has chosen to conceal from others. The degree of disclosure remains a matter of continual negotiation and is to some extent dependent on: the nature of the relationship established; the identity, perceived role and skill of the researcher; and the sense of control, self-esteem and comfort of the respondent.

The perception of harm amongst the respondents themselves may well be different from that of their gatekeepers, or society in general.

To incur the displeasure or sanction of any of these groups is to jeopardize the value of the research findings. The experiences, values, perceptions and agendas of people will vary: the onus is on the researcher to gain insight into the sensitivities of others and minimize the onslaught to such feelings.

To some extent the degree of threat is a matter of personal assessment: what is threatening to one person may be innocuous to another. What a gatekeeper considers sensitive material may not be perceived as such to the person investigating the topic. The challenge is to anticipate how an investigation may be perceived by others, and to build in benefits for those who are willing to participate.

There are, however, commonly accepted social contexts which may lead one to anticipate that certain topics may be especially sensitive. Research in the fields of child abuse, sexual deviance or drug peddling is likely to be fraught with problems of threat and fear of recrimination. On the other hand sometimes seemingly innocuous enquiries can unearth strong threats because of the idiosyncratic experiences of some of the participants that a researcher could not have anticipated; for example, a study of first-time mothers may lead to a respondent disclosing experience of previous abortion or of surrogacy arrangements which to her carry a risk of unwelcome discovery. For this individual, this is a sensitive subject, but the researcher would in all probability have no prior knowledge of such a development.

It sometimes happens that even when sensitivities have been respected the perceived harm exceeds expectations; for example, on occasions a respondent divulges highly sensitive information during the course of an interview with a skilled researcher. The respondent may subsequently regret that 'moment of weakness', and develop hostility towards the person who achieved the disclosure. Where there is a continuing relationship between the two, this can be uncomfortable and inhibiting for both parties. If there is no further contact the respondent can be left with unresolved tensions which may be damaging to self-esteem, confidence or comfort.

Preparation of the researcher

My own experiences as a researcher have exposed me to a number of situations which have involved much heart searching. I am persuaded that there are few black and white answers. Each situation needs to be assessed carefully and minutely. But I believe that researchers are more credible, and perceived as more trustworthy, if they honestly declare the cause of their anxiety and the action taken, rather than covering up the problem that has arisen.

Textbooks on research methods rarely address the reality of such dilemmas. Indeed, as Punch (1986) has commented, such research:

> involves an inexhaustible variety of settings and an endless range of situational exigencies for which ready-made recipes do not exist. The conduct of the researcher, and the outcomes of research, are vulnerable to unique developments in the field and to dramatic predicaments that can often be solved only situationally.

But sweeping the issues under the carpet is not the way to future enlightenment. Every researcher should at least be alive to the issues and prepared in some measure for the decisions and their justification. In the very first piece of research I carried out, I was challenged fairly early into its design to consider what I would do if exactly such situations arose. The investigation involved my going out talking to mothers of very low birth weight babies. The interviews spanned three months after the baby's discharge from a neonatal unit as well as the period of hospitalization. They took place for the most part in the mothers' own homes. My challenger was a psychiatrist on an ethics committee who saw this novice researcher, out in the community, seeing and hearing worrying things, party to burdensome information, and totally unprepared for dealing with it. I was asked, kindly and wisely, to outline my line of communication in such circumstances. On many occasions during the conduct of that study, I had cause to be grateful that I had been forced to address these possibilities from the outset. I have remained indebted to that psychiatrist for his insight and commitment to ensuring that research was not detrimental to the well-being of its subjects or to me, even where the study was exploratory and involved no interventions.

There is a common misperception that only research involving things like radioactive isotopes or experimental interventions really requires ethical approval. This is not so. Even in a study as benign as mine, there was a form of intervention: my presence and my questioning. It had consequences, not as evidently potentially harmful as powerful drugs, maybe, but consequences nonetheless.

Because researchers fear that some areas are too sensitive to research openly, research has occasionally been carried out in a covert way.

Probably the most well known example is Humphrey's (1970) *Tearoom Trade* study of impersonal sex in public places. In this the researcher conducted fieldwork among men having impersonal sex in public facilities. He acted as a 'watch queen'. This enabled him to offer his services as a lookout for intruders, in exchange for the opportunity to observe sexual activity. By means of recording licence numbers of the men's cars, he traced their names and addresses. This enabled him, with changed hairstyle and form of dress, subsequently to visit them at home as part of a 'social health survey'. The richness of data obtained in such a way may be beyond doubt, but many people, myself included, have serious misgivings about the ethics of such deceit (Beauchamp *et al.*, 1982).

Most midwifery research appears innocuous by comparison, but the same rights and ethical principles need to be considered. In fieldwork with certain topics, there seems no way around the predicament that truly informed consent may 'kill many a project stone dead' (Punch, 1986), or be situationally unworkable. Nevertheless, it seems to me, the benefits of knowledge must be most carefully weighed against the consequences to the respondents and those closely associated with them.

However, the fact that certain research studies pose complex ethical problems does not mean that they should not be attempted. As Sieber and Stanley (1988) have argued, some of society's most pressing social questions are those commonly thought to be 'sensitive'. Ignoring them is not a responsible approach to science. Shying away from them simply because they are controversial is also an avoidance of responsibility. But if researchers do embark on such studies, it is imperative that they do not ignore the methodological difficulties inherent in such work (Lee and Renzetti, 1993).

The costs

It is not just to the respondents that harm may accrue. There are considerable costs to be borne by investigators and it must be remembered that 'empirical studies serve not only to create knowledge. They are also the hard currency with which researchers negotiate their careers, and often play an important role in the construction of personal identity and self-esteem' (Frost and Stablein, 1992a).

Researchers themselves may be put at risk because of the nature of their enquiry. Punch (1986) catalogued studies where researchers had been subjected to verbal and physical violence, public caricature, legal challenge, or eviction from the field. There were instances of fieldworkers going insane, panicking or getting cold feet and never embarking on the fieldwork, of 'obstructionist gatekeepers, vacillating sponsors, factionalism in the field setting forcing the researcher to choose sides, organizational resistance, respondents subverting the research role, sexual shenanigans, and disputes about publication and the veracity of findings' (Punch, 1986).

Glazer (1972) analysed the dynamics of many researchers' encounters with respondents, exploring the balance of reciprocity, trust, tolerance, friendship, and identification. Researchers in his accounts were confronted by social injustice, hostility, condemnation, a sense of guilt and other powerful reactions. Against such a backcloth of studies set in dangerous and shadowy social contexts, midwifery research can appear relatively tame and free from problems, but the same issues and conflicts are pertinent nonetheless. Women having babies are part of the wider society.

I have myself had good reason to fear for my personal safety as a result of entering, alone and unprotected, homes where violence was the norm. Working in the field of HIV and AIDS, on occasions I took on board some of the stigma and rejection levelled against those infected with the virus. Psychological damage can be as draining as the fear of physical harm. Painful and alarming disclosures can be extremely wearing. Being told about illegal or immoral actions; seeing behaviours that jeopardize the safety of vulnerable people; being sworn to secrecy about some highly damaging information; all leave the researcher burdened. Personal integrity may be compromised. The strength of one's commitment to scholarly enquiry may be seriously questioned.

I have lost count of the number of times a respondent has said, 'I haven't told another living soul about that'. It can be enormously therapeutic for someone to unburden themselves to a person who says the information disclosed will go no further, but the consequences for the researcher can be onerous. Difficult decisions have to be made. Where do responsibilities begin and end?

Individual responsibility

Since there are often no right answers, it would be unhelpful merely to catalogue points for consideration or to outline a framework for behaviours. Rote learning will only take an individual so far. The unexpected, the perplexing and the threatening situation will still potentially present problems. In order to deal with these well, the researcher needs an understanding of the underlying issues. Arguing the pros and cons for every ethical, legal, professional and practical problem that may arise is beyond the scope of this chapter. Instead, a series of short journeys into real life fieldwork with a sensitive component will be undertaken. No attempt will be made to analyse each situation comprehensively. Rather the illustrations will provide a starting point in the process of considering the arguments and viewpoints. It is important to remember that each individual researcher must be able to give an adequate account of his or her behaviour and defend chosen decisions and actions. It is part of being professionally accountable.

Example 1

Irene was 22 years old, living with her boyfriend, Tom, in a very run down part of a large city. Tom, an unemployed labourer, was the second of three sons. Both his brothers were in prison for crimes of violence – murder and mugging respectively. Irene's own mother refused to visit them at home since she considered the neighbourhood both dangerous and beneath her, but Tom's family dropped in frequently.

Pregnancy was not planned but until 28 weeks was uneventful. Then raised blood pressure necessitated Irene's admission to hospital. An emergency Caesarean section was carried out two weeks later when her pre-eclampsia could not be controlled. The baby girl, Cheryl, weighed 1277 grams and was in good condition at birth, requiring only headbox oxygen. But Irene found the whole experience of having an operation terrifying and was convinced she herself would die.

Her first view of Cheryl was through a haze of drugs and she pronounced her 'quite nice', but once the medication was withdrawn, she was horrified by the child's appearance: she resembled a 'half dead bird' and her mother was revolted. She was extremely loath to touch her. Gradually, over the eight weeks that Cheryl remained in the Neonatal Unit, Irene found she quite enjoyed holding the baby, provided she was well wrapped up in blankets and fast asleep, but awake and crying she terrified her mother. Tom, however, well used to dealing with a stream of small nephews and nieces, appeared quite at home in the Neonatal Unit and handled the baby with pleasure and confidence. This irritated Irene. Her relationship with Tom had always been tempestuous and there were now frequent arguments, on several occasions one or other storming out of the nursery in anger.

Irene saw little of her mother and declared that she had no one to confide in except me. Indeed, she welcomed the opportunity to be involved in a project which gave her ongoing opportunities to talk to someone she perceived to be non-authoritarian. Over the months of her participation in the study, she continued to be preoccupied with the child's 'ugliness', believing there was something very abnormal about her. Medically Cheryl's condition was uncomplicated. Her only problem was a poor toleration of feeds. In real terms to Irene her problems were manifested in excessive vomiting at feed times, the baby going blue in the face and fighting for breath. Perversely, she felt, Cheryl fed beautifully for everyone else.

Such was her terror, that throughout the whole eight weeks, Irene never completed a feed with Cheryl, always passing her on to a neonatal nurse with a variety of excuses why she could not remain in the nursery. But since she believed the nurses had certain expectations of mothers, she took care to use different excuses and apply to different members of staff for help. She considered it would have been quite unacceptable to tell the health care team that she was unwilling to feed her baby. As a researcher, I presented no such threat; she had been assured that I would respect confidences. I gave no advice, and had taken no part in saving the baby's life. As a result she was able to confide that she 'hated' the child and did not want her home.

On my first visit after Cheryl's discharge I found a highly anxious Irene. She and Tom did not go to bed at night but slept uneasily on the floor beside Cheryl's cot. Both were seriously perturbed by her 'screeching', which went on sometimes for as long as five hours. Neither was prepared to be left alone with the baby, fearful that they might harm her if there was no one else to keep them in check.

Against this background, I was more than a little concerned when Irene failed to answer my ring at her door one month after she had taken Cheryl home. The usual repeat visits, after leaving notes through the door, simply established that someone had been into the house between my calls, but there was no word of what had happened to make Irene break our appointment. She had repeatedly discussed with me her hatred towards the baby, and how near she had come to harming her seriously. If her word was true, no one except me knew about this. I felt profoundly troubled.

What was I to do? On the one hand, my contract as a researcher made me respect her confidences. I had given a solemn undertaking to do so. Then too, the quality of my research was at stake. If I intervened I was substantially influencing the situation and any further data collected from her could be invalidated. And how would my clinical colleagues react to 'interference' from outside? They were after all responsible for the health and well-being of this family: I was on their territory. But on the other hand, I was seriously alarmed about the welfare of this child. Was she lying dead in a gas oven? Had Irene also done harm to herself? My responsibility as a human being and as a caring nurse seemed to make it impossible to walk away and do nothing.

The advice of the Ethics Committee proved enormously helpful. They had required me to specify my lines of communication in the event of a situation arising where I was seriously concerned for the welfare of the family. I was able simultaneously to respect the detail of Irene's confidences and to alert the health care team to a potential problem. The agreed course of action was that I phoned my academic supervisor who was a consultant neonatologist. He then rang Irene's GP and asked that the health visitor investigate Irene's absence. I was sufficiently concerned about Irene myself to continue to call, hoping to find her in. My persistence was eventually rewarded. Both mother and baby were alive. The endless screaming had antagonized an elderly neighbour, who had threatened to report the parents to the police for abusing the child. Irene fled to friends' homes. There she abdicated responsibility for bathing and feeding Cheryl, leaving it to her calmer friends. Her flight had helped her to cope, and the passage of time had improved her own ability to look after her larger, more co-ordinated baby.

Example 2

I first became acutely aware of the baggage a researcher brings to any encounter when I was working in the field of HIV and AIDS. Because of its close association with death and sex, there are many sensitivities caught up in this area of practice.

As part of my enquiry I interviewed key professionals throughout the United Kingdom. For one such session I was requested to go to an HIV testing clinic in a large hospital. Finding no signs to this clinic, I approached the staff in an ordinary outpatient clinic for advice. I was totally unprepared for their reaction. Not only did they not know, but they did not *want* to know. They referred me to another building. In all five encounters I had with staff in different departments in that hospital in the course of my search for the clinic, I felt the same sense of discomfort. I met with outright scorn, conspiratorial whispering, and public humiliation. My failure to state the purpose of my visit began as an accident, but became deliberate. Much as I smarted under the reactions, it gave me a salutary experience akin to that of a patient attending for testing for the first time. But unlike them, I was hundreds of miles from my home, extremely unlikely to meet anyone I knew, and not actually seeking a test. Nonetheless, it was still a painful experience.

When I eventually arrived in the clinic I was directed to take a seat at the back of the room. It soon became apparent that I was in the presence of rows of prostitutes. In the short wait for my respondent, I had an opportunity to analyse my own reactions. I realized the prejudices and attitudes I had held (but had not recognized previously) could potentially jeopardize the quality of the data I was collecting in this sensitive area. As a consequence, I subsequently attempted to cultivate a heightened awareness and alertness, consciously developing an approach which was sensitive to the needs of respondents of different persuasions, orientations and beliefs.

As part of this preparation I became much more aware of the use of language. In the world of HIV and AIDS, words and expressions in common usage may acquire totally different connotations. Common assumptions about gender, affiliations and attitudes may all be misplaced. At times my own value systems were competing with those of my respondents. It was impossible to become cognizant of all such differences and pitfalls in the space of a few weeks, but in recognizing my own *naïveté*, I was better able to recognize the pitfalls, and avoid some of the mistakes. It was still difficult internally to deal with the accounts of blatant discrimination and injustice and insensitive management of individuals, but I was more aware of my own reactions and the effect I might have on respondents and on the data.

Indeed, to some extent, being brought face to face with my own attitudes and feelings helped me to understand what respondents talked about in disclosing their own problems in this area. I knew what interviewees, who were also health care professionals, meant when they talked about being offended by shock tactics, being discomposed by blatant references to unusual sexual practices, being ambivalent about accepting an invitation to a client's home; feeling that they were being asked to condone everything. For those clinicians whose experience has been extensive and who have developed a special skill in this area, it can be difficult to identify with the new recruit for whom this seems like a disturbing and dangerous world, but their perspective is legitimate too, and in-depth discussions with specialists helped me to keep a balance and to understand their world.

This was the first research I had carried out in an area of practice with which I was not familiar clinically. There are problems as well as benefits in entering a sensitive field as a novice. Although I had read extensively on the subject and talked to specialists informally as well as on working parties, it was possible I would simply fail to understand what was being said. I might inadvertently offend or upset respondents because I was unaware of the nuances of this speciality. On the other hand, I was able to ask for explanations of the obvious. I could probe for understanding of the taken-for-granted things, which a more expert clinician could not do with any degree of credibility.

Because of all the potential problems, care needed to be taken to verify the truth of the study findings. An important part of the design of this enquiry involved testing the results with a variety of groups of people to be confident that an accurate and scientific analysis was achieved. Opportunities were built in to enable practitioners, educators, managers, and clients to discuss the results and determine whether they represented the real world as they perceived it. I repeatedly checked my interpretations against the yardstick of experience.

Example 3

Asking clinicians about their practices and beliefs in relation to withholding or withdrawing treatment from extremely sick neonates was guaranteed to be emotionally taxing. This is a difficult environment to enter. The tensions and stresses of staff working in intensive care units are well documented. I found myself caught more than once in emotional crossfire about which I could only dimly discern the causes. When I was intent on cultivating trust and building up rapport with the medical and nursing staff, I found it disconcerting to feel the tensions even when they actually stemmed from administrative problems or personality clashes. It was all too easy to take them personally. There was too a very real danger of over-identification with respondents which I had to keep to the forefront of my mind.

Nor was the nature of the subject an easy one to explore. There were many sensitivities wrapped up in its boundaries. A number of clinicians have already experienced the trauma of being taken to court by parents who hold a grievance against them for the death or impaired life of their child. Legal backing appears uncertain. Furthermore, media programmes designed to bring these matters to public attention do little to reassure clinicians. There are threats inherent in asking them to share their experiences on such delicate matters.

Methodologically, much careful thought was needed in the design of this project. I considered it was important to spend time establishing trust in each unit before interviewing staff. Part of this preparation involved my being present at all hours of the day and night, at weekends, as well as public holidays. Words were chosen carefully: 'euthanasia' was avoided. Respondents were encouraged to detail their own experiences of specific cases to give them a sense of control and confidence in their own coherence. Access to staff and the selection of representative respondents was carried out in careful conjunction with the practitioners and in line with clinical commitments and demands. But for me, there was a price to be paid. I was a visitor in close knit teams: an outsider. I had to be vigilant, not to overstep the bounds of my welcome. The dividing line between involvement and intrusion required repeated testing.

And there was a heavy weight to be carried emotionally in conducting an enquiry which involved interviewing many professionals. It was burdensome to be in receipt of frequent stories involving powerful emotions. These included not only those involving neonates, but also accounts of the deaths of close relatives, the burdens of handicap and the stress of life events of various kinds. Some of these touched glancingly on my own raw nerves which I had thought were healed. An important feature of in-depth interviewing is that the researcher needs to concentrate totally throughout the discussion, weaving in past information and taking account of additional and serendipitous keys to the respondent's feelings and views. But this requires a clarity of thinking and a freedom from distraction. It is vital to come to each encounter with a freshness and keen interest in what this new individual will contribute to understanding of this topic.

I quickly learned that being up half the night, and working long stretches without a break, dulled my senses. I had to limit the number of interviews I conducted concurrently. I had to forget my pride in my own ability to survive a gruelling schedule and learn to be kinder to myself. Only that way could I give what was needed to each research encounter. In previous studies where profound emotions had been exposed, I had nominated colleagues to listen to what burdened me and thereby rid myself of tensions which could inhibit effective future interviewing. With this enquiry the information received was of a greater sensitivity. I had given careful assurances to all those involved that I would do all in my power to safeguard the identity of each institution as well as each individual. A sense of absolute safety was vital to the success of the enquiry. I had to learn to deal with the psychological burden using inner resources and relaxing outside pursuits. However, much of the time spent data collecting, I was away from home and my usual sources of refreshing. New techniques had to be developed; other outlets for tension found.

Some fundamentals

These few examples are merely illustrative of the reality of researching in sensitive areas. As Glazer (1972) expressed it:

> The satisfactions, excitement, frustrations, challenges, and agonies of field research are not time bound. They are as real and relevant today as when they occurred.... The questions continue to be fundamental ... crucial and must be constantly expressed, discussed and evaluated. Those who would participate in the adventures of research must continually confront the most challenging questions of scientific ethics and social responsibility. For we are deeply 'involved in mankind'.

Health care professionals are the envy of many other researchers. An enormously rich field for enquiry is open to them, and they are, indeed 'deeply involved in mankind.' Where they understand intimately the nuances of the situations they are investigating, they can bring special skills and an extra dimension to both data collection and analysis. On occasions there may be a conflict between the demands of academia and professional instinct. But a primary loyalty towards the greater good of the population served by the health care service should be sufficient motivation to compel them to examine the research endeavour, and move towards more openness and honesty.

Although definitive answers to any dilemma are elusive, there are certain fundamental prerequisites relating to respect for respondents and responsible stewardship of data, as the previous chapter has outlined (see also Beauchamp et al., 1982; Boruch and Cecil, 1983; Punch, 1986; Hunt, 1989; Frost and Stablein, 1992b; Lee and Renzetti, 1993; Sieber, 1993). Careful thought must be given to the design and conduct of the enquiry, to the fieldwork experience, to the analysis of the data, and to the dissemination of findings. At all levels, sensitivities may be offended and quality jeopardized. Awareness of the issues and rehearsal of the options may go some way towards minimizing any harm.

I share the view of Punch (1986) that 'openness, debate, individual responsibility, and professional accountability on the conduct of research are more likely to spell out a sensible and healthy approach to the moral dilemmas in fieldwork than regulation.'

Codes tend to be too vague and may indeed create unnecessary barriers. Rigid standards and sanctions cannot be imposed in a world where there are no clearly definable ways of calculating costs and benefits. Research ethics are not clear-cut matters which conform to such laws or guidelines, but open debate of the issues can both take account of fundamental principles and allow for the vagaries of specific situations. Coming clean about the realities of fieldwork experience may well go some way towards achieving a greater integrity.

Acknowledgements

I am indebted to Kenneth Boyd and Jennifer Sleep for their helpful comments on the first draft of this chapter.

References

Beauchamp, T. L., Faden, R. R., Wallace, R. J. Jr and Walters, L. (eds). (1982). *Ethical Issues in Social Science Research*. John Hopkins University Press.

Boruch, R. F. and Cecil, J. S. (1983). *Solutions to Ethical and Legal Problems in Social Research*. Academic Press.

Frost, P. J. and Stablein, R. E. (1992a). Lessons from the journeys. In *Doing Exemplary Research* (P. J. Frost and R. E. Stablein, eds), pp. 270–292, Sage.

Frost, P. J. and Stablein, R. E. (eds). (1992b). *Doing Exemplary Research*. Sage.

Glazer, M. (1972). *The Research Adventure: Promise and Problems of Field Work*. Random House.

Humphreys, L. (1970). *Tearoom Trade: Impersonal Sex in Public Places*. Aldine.

Hunt, J. C. (1989). *Psychoanalytic Aspects of Fieldwork*. Sage.

Kelman, H. C. (1982). Ethical issues in different social science methods. In *Ethical Issues in Social Science Research* (T. L. Beauchamp, R. R. Faden, R. J. Wallace Jr and L. Walters, eds), pp. 40–98. Johns Hopkins University Press.

Lee, R. M. and Renzetti, C. M. (1993). The problems of researching sensitive topics: An overview and Introduction. In *Researching Sensitive Topics* (C. M. Renzetti and R. M. Lee, eds), pp. 3–13. Sage.

MacIntyre, A. (1982). Risk, harm, and benefit assessment as instruments of moral evaluation. In *Ethical Issues in Social Science Research*. (T. L. Beauchamp, R. R. Faden, R. J. Wallace Jr and L. Waters, eds), pp. 175–189. John Hopkins University Press.

Mitchell, R. G. Jr (1991). Secrecy and disclosure in fieldwork. In *Experiencing Fieldwork: An Insider View of Qualitative Research* (W. B. Shaffir and R. A. Stebbins, eds), pp. 97–108. Sage.

Punch, M. (1986). *The Politics and Ethics of Fieldwork*. Sage.

Sieber, J. E. (1993). The ethics and politics of sensitive research. In *Researching Sensitive Topics* (C. M. Renzetti and R. M. Lee, eds), pp. 14–26. Sage.

Sieber, J. E. and Stanley, B. (1988). Ethical and professional dimensions of socially sensitive research. *Am. Psychol.*, **43**, 49–55.

Index